Cross Training

How to Train Smarter to Become a Better Runner

(A Long-distance Runner's Guide to Weight-lifting and Cross-training)

Paul Riddle

Published By **Cathy Nedrow**

Paul Riddle

Cross Training: How to Train Smarter to Become a Better Runner (A Long-distance Runner's Guide to Weight-lifting and Cross-training)

ISBN   978-1-7776010-4-1

No part of this guidebook shall be reproduced in any form without permission in writing from the publisher except in the case of brief quotations embodied in critical articles or reviews.

Legal & Disclaimer

The information contained in this book is not designed to replace or take the place of any form of medicine or professional medical advice. The information in this book has been provided for educational & entertainment purposes only.

The information contained in this book has been compiled from sources deemed reliable, and it is accurate to the best of the Author's knowledge; however, the Author cannot guarantee its accuracy and validity and cannot be held liable for any errors or omissions. Changes are periodically made to this book. You must consult your doctor or get professional medical advice before using any of the suggested remedies, techniques, or information in this book.

Table Of Contents

Chapter 1: Cross Training Components and Features

Weightlifting

It has now turned out to be essential to preserve a robust, strong frame. This undeniably well-known sample has made human beings cognizance closer on their real trends and has made them privy to the importance of right fitness.

People presently spend first-rate cash on weightlifting structures to accomplish the real frame they have got constantly desired for.

Men and women each have come to understand that weightlifting received 't simply cause them to sound but in addition reason them to look amazing and further boom the manner the arena sees them. Individuals are looking for the best techniques to lose their abundance fat and get the appropriate frame shape.

They make investments a ton of time, energy and coins to form their our our bodies and hold on with a higher life. Weightlifting structures can likewise defend humans from a ton of clinical problems, making the coronary coronary heart, lungs, and liver extra grounded and higher and furthermore their cerebrums extra alert.

Weightlifting did inside the proper way and the proper sum, following all insurances and strategies, someone with dedication can in the long run accomplish the proper body type and physical health.

To arrive at their aim actual look, people usually be part of exercise centers, wherein they're given a huge scope of proficient weight lifting device to help them with growing their our bodies. There are likewise coaches present to assist them in doing the right sports in the right manner so their exercise routine gives the fantastic and maximum proficient results.

The running shoes provide the person with their professional opinion in order that the man or woman is familiar with right procedures and makes certain that over exertion does not display up. Equipment like dumbbells, heavy balls, treadmills, cycles, and so on. Are available inside the gymnasium and people can use the device that fits their exercising regime.

However, there are individuals who, due to their busy artwork schedules and special elements are not able to be a part of a health club and construct the frame that they discover extremely good. In such cases, they should purchase the device they require from severa retail stores

which might be on hand everywhere and anywhere.

Make certain you advocate a expert and an consuming habitual expert close by weightlifting. This will assist you with arranging out a valid exercising recurring with a purpose to show effective in reinforcing and fostering your frame the right manner. Follow valid strategies, play it constant, and hold up together with your workout habitual and you'll accomplish the frame which you usually preferred.

Gymnastics

If you are eager on aerobatic, you may want to have a decent jogging facts on the tumbling hardware that you will utilize. Since that may be a especially brilliant difficulty depend, it's miles superb to end up familiar with the overall instructions and everyday machine.

One such piece of hardware is the equilibrium pillar. There are many minor departure from this, but the real shaft is some factor comparable. It is a couple inches massive, and they come in 8' or 10' lengths. For novices, an exercising middle may additionally have a pillar that simply sits a couple creeps over the floor. Even and lopsided bars are one greater conspicuous piece of hardware for a wonderful many people. While the ones are numerous bits of gadget, the talents required for them are comparable.

Vaulting hardware is vital, but as it isn't with the useful aid of and massive on the center of interest, it has a bent to be not noted decently without any problem. But there are numerous varieties of vaulting tool. Springboards are the maximum notably recognized. Vaulting portions are applied pair with certainly one of a kind bits of aerobatic device.

Landing mats are one extra huge piece of hardware that is mostly a component-word. Without the valid mats, gymnasts could be simply harmed in the route of a every day workout. The mats ought to be business enterprise to the point of allowing the competitor to nail their end, however sensitive enough to ingest the effect in their touchdown.

Rings and identical bars are or three types of acrobatic equipment which might be usually implemented. These are each within the

Olympics but are basically used by men. Practically any kind of acrobatic machine is made for the two grown-u.S. Of americaand youngsters. The factors could be precise, as will the fitness safeguards. There is probably considerably greater cushioning on kids' gadget.

Any acrobat need to have a ton of sensible dexterity, and feature the selection to bypass judgment on exactly how a good deal exertion they will be setting right into a circulate. An immoderate quantity of exertion and they're obligated to foul their flip or overshoot their imprint. Too little exertion and they will skip over the mark. Either condition is at risk to result in a bodily problem. It have to all of the time be remembered that tumbling are hard to do effectively, and an character can severely damage themselves assuming they project to make use of any acrobatic gear without valid making equipped. Even professional gymnasts must no longer workout consultation with out a person spotting them.

Cardio

The purpose for cardiovascular sports is to decorate and broaden your coronary coronary heart, work your lungs and in addition increase route, blood flow, and respiratory capability. These additives cooperate to border your cardiovascular 'framework.' Accordingly, the essential gain of aerobic making prepared is to further expand your frame's cardiovascular framework via making geared up it to art work greater successfully.

What is the great aerobic exercise?

This reaction is perhaps the most truthful simply one in every of all, and also you probably ought to have a tough time believing it when you pay hobby it. Basically, the excellent cardio exercise you can ever perform for your whole existence is the fine that you DO! What we're announcing here is that you do not want to waste time quite some time trying every new cardio utility or every new shape of aerobic training that comes alongside. You'd be nice served by using manner of the use of making an investment your electricity DOing the genuine exercise.

What are the extraordinary aerobic sports sports to do at domestic?

Obviously, in all likelihood the least demanding method for getting into a first rate cardio workout is to take a stroll in reality. But recollect to walk quick sufficient to preserve that coronary coronary heart fee up! Alternatively, you could flow for a run as nicely. Assuming you're efficiently fortunate to approach a pool, you can go for a plunge, actually make sure you are doing laps!

Chapter 2: Paleo Fanatics and Foods

That Ruin Your Life The disturbing element approximately any fanatic is no matter how unpalatable they will be these days, one month from now they will be a fan and unsightly near something one-of-a-kind.

If you've got were given run over broadly instructing books, you presumably have understood that I generally check a modified Paleo diet. At the point when I say adjusted, I say that is for the cause that I don't clearly adhere to every one of the suggestions set via using the distinctly logical Paleo humans institution. Assuming you want to, that approves of me. A huge detail parents select out Paleo to get a extra streamlined body and to experience better. It has been showed that you may do this, even following the Paleo food regimen about 80% of the time. Furthermore allow's be sincere, assuming we set irrational expectancies for ourselves, we obtained't ever adhere to any weight loss plan. A respectable ingesting ordinary wants to artwork with having the choice to squeeze right into a really normal manner of life.Does the ones Paleo fan disguise away a ways from everyone else? Do they no longer stress a vehicle? I'm glad to record, you could get in shape and sense better with the Paleo diet plan, and also you don't want to be a Paleo fanatic.

I expect the facts about the Paleo time is interesting. I take delivery of there is a ton of truth about it. In any case, allow's be honest, that became quite a while inside the past, and there may be a ton of hypothesis. So the mountain guy component isn't genuinely crucial to me. Be that as it may, results are critical. I referenced in advance than that there are techniques for following the Paleo weight-reduction plan. You can follow it a hundred%, or you may comply with it extra frequently than now not. Furthermore the two of them paintings. In the occasion which you are experiencing an immune device hassle, you want to examine it a hundred percent. Assuming however, you're in reality seeking to lose muscle to fats ratio and revel in a fantastic deal improved, extra often than no longer Paleo will flip out first rate for you. So it isn't the stone age man exposure that requests to me. What clearly does talk to me is that Paleo appears OK and assists many humans with getting more in shape, and revel in better? How does Paleo do this? I'm a surely unfavorably inclined type man or woman, and I will try to make clear this in primary phrases. I'm now not a consultant or researcher, but rather I without a doubt have gleaned a few giant experience about allergy over the years.

It is a reality. Many humans agencies our bodies try to avoid grains, dairy, and extraordinary proteins. Hypersensitivities are the our bodies response to these things it doesn't like. These topics are in huge part strong proteins. The component outcomes are the outcome of the body attempting to defend itself from proteins it doesn't talk in self assurance to. All in all, even as you are furnished to three difficulty your body doesn't like, it is largely saying, there can be this protein I don't apprehend approximately. It should be a parasite or microbe that is trying to

purpose me damage, so I will attempt to kill it. Presently that is probable an exciting approach for putting it, but this is the allergy essentially (appreciably). So the frame attempts to kill this thing that it thinks can be a parasite, or microorganism or other attacking substance. It discharges huge masses of artificial substances to remove it. These encompass histamine, cortisol, and others. Your guard framework implies business enterprise. So what takes vicinity is a state of affairs of contamination from the start. Something might be angry. Assuming it's dirt and your nose, your sinus sections may be annoyed and enlarged. In the most pessimistic situation conditions, your body is assaulting itself. It is hurting itself with all due respect, and that is the crucial concept of immune gadget troubles.

Hay fever is an disturbing immune system condition, but it's far actually innocent. On the off chance that this situation takes some one-of-a-kind shape, you can have diabetes or different proper and detrimental, fitness troubles. Truly, the big majority that have meals hypersensitivities are oversensitive to similar kinds of proteins. Furthermore reflect onconsideration on what they will be? Generally grains and dairy, soy and veggies. Indeed, that is a popular problem for a few people with sensitivities. But even if you do now not have allergies which you recognize of, those proteins may additionally furthermore nevertheless cause responses from your frame. Many people hold ingesting subjects which is probably slowly killing them or at splendid, making their lifestyles depressing and high-priced. You might have been consuming meals sorts because of the fact a youngster which might be inflicting aggravation in your body. I understand, I speak as a count number of fact. But the good information is whilst you eliminate the ones property of irritation, the inflammation calms down, and also you experience better.

But that isn't all. It has been tested typically, which grains carbs and sugars are moreover making us fat. Food additives are as properly. Additives had been related to massive infections like coronary coronary heart conditions and pretty intellectual problems like dementia. So that is the piece of Paleo that I love.

You will preserve on seeing critiques approximately wheat and unique grains and the manner they're connected to diabetes and exceptional diseases. It is a fact, which Paleo is the right eating everyday for almost all people, and could carry great effects. So mountain guy or no cavern occupant, that is an consuming ordinary that assessments out and brings results. It doesn't make any distinction in the event which you name it Paleo or Caveman food plan, what's important is this is the ingesting routine we ought to be following to appearance outstanding and sense superb. Paleo thru using some exclusive name.

Nutrition for Cross Training

Paleo and Cross Training are often applied collectively. It's obviously actual that you may enhance consequences with consuming lots much less energy through working towards too. You will decorate effects with an interest time desk, with the aid of which incorporates an low cost consuming normal. Diet and workout are purported to cooperate to keep properly being and energy.

Cross Training is an interest framework created at a few degree within the years with the resource of Coach Greg Glassman. It is both a commercial employer framework provided in severa fitness centers and a framework that you could do all by myself. It includes continuously evolving immoderate recognition practices more often than no longer, with loads. It is a utilitarian form of interest in that the schedules depend on everyday tendencies. For example, a Cross

Training hobby can also additionally involve similar muscle groups and improvement as searching after something on a excessive rack. Extreme popularity practices like Cross Training have substantiated themselves as amazing fat eliminators. It is smarter to do an interesting activity energetically for a quick time frame than to do a similar exercise over and another time for a in reality long term. When you get your digestion up thru way of doing an immoderate awareness exercising session, the body maintains on consuming fats after the hobby is completed. More fat eating appreciably quicker. It consumes fatter taking walks energetically for a quick time frame than strolling little by little for big stretches. The regular Cross Training exercise calls for 2 minutes to thirty minutes to execute. Broadly teaching can be an excessive preparing for weight lifters or a more easygoing technique for nicely being and rehabilitation.

If you need to get more familiar with Cross Training or attempt part of the sports activities sports, you may do as such through touring CrossFit.Com. Broadly teaching shows truly one in every of weight manipulate plans, the Paleo weight-reduction plan, and the place, contingent upon your objectives. By far maximum of Cross mentors, likewise look at the Paleo diet plan. Broadly teaching humans are eager on getting but plenty strength as also can want to moderately be predicted from their food. They do that thru which include more sturdy fat like nuts and olives to their eating regimens. This works in impeccably with the Paleo food plan. They upload all of the greater low glycemic meals assets in choice to higher glycemic meals sorts like most carbs. Broadly coaching abilties admirably with Paleo in moderate of the truth that with Paleo you in all fact do get to devour a awesome deal of food. You can eat severa more modest dinners throughout the day. Both Paleo and Cross Training address meals as gas for the body.

Either the Paleo food regimen or Cross getting prepared will supply effective results. Doing every as a direction for dwelling will get the great outcomes minimum measure of time. Both Paleo and Cross Training must be viable all on my own and your terms.

Benefits Of Cross Training For Cyclists

What is substantially teaching and how can it feature? How can it art work?

When you partake in any excessive-depth recreation, your coronary coronary heart can't understand sports activities sports. This is considering the fact that the coronary heart in reality sees 'how difficult you are functioning' and may't determine what recreation you're doing.

So, you could do quite plenty any immoderate-depth recreation and get"for the most element healthy." However, your leg muscle tissue, alternatively, need to regulate"explicitly" to the sport you're doing. For example, at the off chance which you do running, your muscle organizations will modify to on foot. But because you are on foot and no longer cycling, you'll find "cycling particular muscle health" will drop off drastically.

We can sum up then that significantly educating constructs modern well being through doing numerous video video video games, however realise that assuming you do diverse video games continuously, your precise cycling health will vanish. Is doing extensively teaching counter-intuitive?

The way to fruitful broadly education is in reality to keep a bit biking taking place the grounds which you can as an possibility no longer lose ALL your high-quality cycling properly-being you've built up.

Maintaining more than one rides seven days is to the factor of retaining your muscles adjusted to biking, while you extend 'enormous fitness' collectively collectively with your unique excessive-depth video video games. This is the manner to effectively carrying out flow-schooling.

But what's the point of doing broadly teaching assuming I lose some biking fitness?

If you've completed a complete summer season of cyclosportives or visiting or definitely been on your bicycle constantly the entire summer season, then, at that element, it is the appropriate possibility for a mental wreck.

Building up leisurely like this with the aid of requiring a few investment out from all three hundred and sixty 5 days cycling, implies you come healthy and rejuvenated prepared to position extra accentuation on your cycle making geared up while you're prepared. Preferably, you can instead now not be one degree of health lasting through the 12 months: you want to amplify your health to multiple tops in the course of the biking summer time, no longer over Christmas!

Moreover, widely teaching can help with fortifying bones and muscle mass you don't use in cycling. For example, on foot, taking walks, mountain climbing and exercise middle paintings is weight bearing and might help with fortifying your bones, preserving off osteoporosis, a few issue greater cyclists have to recognize approximately, mainly ladies.

Some considered one in all a kind times of high-depth video games you may undergo in thoughts are crosscountry skiing, swimming, route running, snow-shoeing, inline skating, and paddling. Consider mountain trekking at the off hazard that you've been out and approximately throughout the late spring. You'll be submersed in nature, make bigger terrific leg fortitude and be far from road visitors.

Know that there may be an expectation to take in information to the ones games and you want to start slow while your frame adjusts to the fashionable exercising. Final terms:

The key take-domestic thing proper right here is that glide-schooling permits you to be clearly healthy and revitalized over a few months while the ones who've been using their motorcycles all wintry climate will maximum probable be displaying symptoms and symptoms of tiredness and boredom.

So, have a first rate break, respect new video games and expect a few close to domestic great rides three hundred and sixty five days from now even as the pleasant of the climate and your health coincide!

Chapter 3: Cross Training for Runners

A Recipe for Efficient Running

Those who run longer distances frequently use protein powder arrangements or a dinner substitution powder speedy preceding to getting geared up or dashing, as those are less hard to machine than wealthy suppers earlier than a run. Just as adequate hydration, regular sprinters generally supplement their consuming regimens with most cancers prevention stores and a high-quality multivitamin supplement to assist with keeping up with electricity degrees and tissue recovery. Be that as it could, glaringly, weight

loss plan by myself, big for what it's properly properly well worth, isn't good enough. It may additionally astonish numerous sprinters to find out that running by myself isn't the crucial kind of hobby. The evidence is aggregating that walking exhibition may be drastically advanced by way of the usage of manner of broadly education - increasing one's displaying execution to technique for diverse video games or workout applications further to beating the street or the route.
Cross Training and Injury Prevention

For most walking opposition who extensively teach, the leader clarification they test with for their non-compulsory workout is harm counteraction. There are severa high-quality benefits, but it deserves investigating how considerably teaching can help with forestalling wounds. As veteran sprinters understand, the majority of the injuries they land up nursing are introduced approximately through abuse and mileage. Rather than considering these as certainties, in any case, a superior method is to think about their motives and check whether or not or now not there are pragmatic remedy plans and precaution techniques.

Many opposition dread that resting will spark off a discount in properly-being, which is basically now not the situation. Broadly educating can dispose of the pressure from the joints and muscle tissues which have been set underneath pressure inside the direction of the run and keep up with cardiovascular fitness, truely as increasing the energy of middle muscle corporations inside the direction of the decrease decrease again and mid-vicinity

essential for maintaining up with right stance and limiting in addition harm. Weight-getting ready or swimming are both first-rate techniques of soothing sore joints even as developing fortitude and versatility on the equal time as assisting pinnacle wellbeing and shielding the body from the effect mileage coming approximately due to walking-just exercise exercises.

Cross Training and Injury Recovery

To stay with regards to harm highly longer: widely instructing may be extremely important in improving from harm. A few wounds require restraint from strolling assuming there can be to be any shot at restoration; appreciably teaching can guide fitness and successfully help the harmed tissue with enhancing. This is the region in which on foot-big sports activities sports and machine could make their mark. Water is walking, the cardiovascular exercise conveyed through way of the curved device (which suits

better and decrease frame utilising strolling improvement with out the impact) and inline skating are amazing substitutes for taking walks.

Enhancing Efficiency

There are some high-quality benefits to keep in mind also. Maybe the most attractive to sprinters is that broadly training enables boost up with the aid of manner of increasing electricity and productiveness. Broadly teaching offers time past regulation, not plenty much less, to be spent walking out, however on physical video games a good way to beautify cardiovascular health without harming joints and destroying muscle filaments. The final results is that the character is in higher actual shape for a race that might be capability with running-definitely sports.

Mobilizing Motivation

Another concept is the high first-class, propelling influences of extensively coaching. Sprinters run thinking about the fact that they like it; but most will concede that there are instances at the same time as comparable schedules, similar streets, and trails, can alternate into pretty stupid. Going for a run feeling exhausted or irritated might be no longer going to assist the competitor in getting the quality enjoy the exercise. Enhancing strolling with non-obligatory significantly teaching practices gives series, restoring concept and assisting cardiovascular well being simply as improving muscle energy.

Active Recovery

A in addition highlight bear in mind is the critical method of dynamic healing workout after a run. This isn't to indicate a whole abrogation of relaxation periods following a run. Rest stays important to keeping up with perfect health; in any case, a slight dynamic healing workout at the same time as acted inside the initial hours following an workout empowers the competitor to carry out an essentially major healing over honest resting.

Fitness During the Off-season

For a few sprinters, the slow time of 3 hundred and sixty 5 days length gives precise hardships. To run or no longer to run - this is the hassle! Running without restoration and relaxation may be counterproductive, prompting an glaringly greater awful large presentation next season, not a superior one. The slow time of yr is the vicinity in which progressed broadly coaching should make its mark. This doesn't propose an entire suspension of strolling, but it can permit absolute relaxation located thru hockey, ball, swimming, curved making geared up, cycling, masses, yoga, even hand at hand stopping. Any of these (or a mix of a few) can allow the frame to get over ultimate season's abuse wounds and maintain up with top health.

The Verdict

There is a large scope of substantially teaching options to browse, and it's miles important to re-underscore that they're no longer predicted to supplant strolling because the essential exercising yet to enhance and beautify it. But runners who need to prevent harm or get higher because it have to be from an gift damage, or who want to decorate their motivation to teach, or to boost their overall performance and tempo at on foot, need to start to skip raining with out similarly take away.

Have You Checked Out the Cross Training Possibilities to Burn Fat Yet?

Being an character from the weight loss phase locations you solidly in advance than the most extensively recognized "reproduction fats regimens." You see them in talents at the net, in magazines and concentrate individuals analyzing them in speak. Be that as it is able to, have you ever thoroughly taken into consideration it to discover what you need?

Gym artwork

out Aerobic

workout

Calorie

counting

Dieting

Right? All things taken into consideration, manifestly. It is legitimate. These famous modalities contend with enterprise, be that as it may, they may be b-o-r-I-n-g. Along the ones traces, it is structured upon you to think outside the significantly diagnosed weight loss subject. Think great feeding food and a laugh wearing occasions. How prolonged has it been since you sustained your body with one or the alternative meals or motion? Possibly as far as feasible lower back to 6th grade? Maybe. OK. Here is the association. Your lifestyles has emerge as excessively unsurprising. For that purpose you are carrying the extra layers of fats. Since you are exhausted crazy. The time has come to step it up. End your existence to a higher degree. Your body too.

There are some tremendous food sorts you are preserving off near your every day supper prep with a view that will help you with finishing the fat consume art work. Think antioxidant.

Chapter 3: Cross Training for Basketball

It is pretty obvious that hobby continues advancing at speedy stages; Access to better device, more education device, electricity and conditioning, fitness center time, summer season leagues, spring leagues, elite leagues, camps, and so on. This increase in get proper of get admission to to to sources, in my view, has delivered on greater issues than blessings. Youth are in reality being specialised earlier into their recreation and function. This has induced increasingly more gamers to burn out, and we are seeing increasing numbers of basketball game enthusiasts with overuse accidents.

According to Canada Basketball's Long Term Athlete Development Model (LTAD), every engine development direction I took through University, and the demanding measure of examination: WE ARE SPECIALIZING OUR ATHLETES TOO EARLY! Our ball kids want to create and consummate ALL engine designs, further to the ones specific to b-ball. As I might see it, the whole thing element we are capable of manipulate for our children permits them to research an collection of bodily video games and sports (Cross Training). This series allows them to address severa engine designs (so we paintings on development in preferred) but further permits our early life to grow to be capable in various settings.

The blessings of appreciably educating include improvement all of the time, lessening the shot at injury, execution enhance, and lowering competitor drop/located on out. We actually need to keep our b-ball opposition sound, drew in, and acting tremendous at the court. To that surrender I felt the Steve Nash Training Day Commercial is so pertinent to b-ball and the importance of Cross Training. Steve Nash is one of the maximum expert competition within the NBA who LOVES what he does, is exceptional at an series of sports activities sports sports, and has a awesome time doing it. I acquire as true with Steve Nash's affiliation in substantially education, as a teen and teen, assumes a vital aspect in his prosperity and existence span as a ball athlete.

It is our goal as strength specialists, mentors, volunteers, guardians, and allies to present our b-ball competition a legitimate climate to recognise! Assuming your teen likes ball, they will go along with the glide in the course of b-ball as they get extra mounted. Early specialization for our adolescence will lower their presentation, vocation existence span, and notice them in threat of damage. We need to induce our formative years to strive soccer, lacrosse, baseball, tune, and lots of others.

At Prehab we apprehend the importance of creating development designs first. We recognise the importance of consummating development. What we do in recent times, may not be explicit to b-ball, but is vital for the b-ball competitor's drawn out development. Broadly teaching thoroughly can be the presentation improve tool you have got been seeking out!

Dancing is a Great Form of Cross Training For Runners Cross making ready for sprinters can really be extended outdoor of the domain names of taking walks, weight lifting, bicycling and swimming. One form of circulate education

that maximum sprinters don't keep in mind and that I might probably want to talk approximately is dancing.

Dancing can be masses of a laugh, and absolutely everyone that has performed it constantly can endure witness to that it has a tendency to be a hint of exertions too. Obviously, a splendid many people don't understand how a superb deal paintings moving can be thinking about the truth that it's miles a ton like ice skating. Early traditional dance examples gained't depart you all that sweat-soaked or tired, but as you enhance, you may save you a whole lot much less frequently for steering and will task extra convoluted actions that permits you to require extra strength and patience. Moving the night time time away is an brilliant method for ingesting some power on the identical time as appreciating yourself.

One of the finest blessings that transferring has over unique forms of substantially teaching is that it's miles an terrific motion to address your equilibrium. For a outstanding many humans, transferring might be commonly a cardiovascular action and obtained't located an entire lot of weight on your legs or decrease again. You don't have to be searching terrific to realise it. You will in reality want to artwork your muscle mass in an sudden way in evaluation to common, and could better observe each foot/eye and hand/eye coordination. Moving is a motion that is first-class presented with others, but it have to likewise be feasible popular overall performance. You can also additionally want to hit the dance ground with outsiders, or depend upon the style you may hit the dance ground without or with everyone else. A few styles of shifting require extra region than others, however commonly, you may oversee thoroughly to your living room or out of doors.

If you live in a metropolitan place, there will most possibly be some clubs which might be open on the ends of the week if no longer within the route of the week. Dance studios also can likewise have a dance hall and latin moving night time one time in line with week or while usually on pinnacle in their vast examples to exit now and again. You might probable truly have the choice to discover a few close by corridors which have dance evenings on a few not unusual agenda. My advice is to find out a associate, take a few instructions, and exit and experience yourself. Simply maintain in thoughts in order no longer to consume or drink excessively while you're out having a amazing time or you may find out that the shifting is all the more an responsibility in choice to a bonus in your broadly teaching. Then all all over again, if you are having sufficient fun, then maybe you may not! Chapter eleven:

Recipes

Breakfast

Recipes

Paleo Crepes

Ingredients

Coconut flour – 2 tbsp. Eggs – 2 large

Coconut oil – 1 tbsp. Melted Water – ½ cup

Coconut milk – 2 tbsp. For cooking

Method

1. In a meals processor, beat collectively the eggs and coconut flour.

2. Add water and 1 tbsp. Coconut oil and heartbeat till blended nicely.

3. In a 8-inch skillet, warm temperature 1 tsp. Coconut oil over medium-low warm temperature.

4. Pour ¼-cup hitter onto the skillet and spread to the rims of the pan.

five. Cook until bubbles form, then, at that thing, flip and put together dinner dinner the opportunity aspect. Around four to five mins desired.

6. Transfer the crepe to a plate.

7. Repeat the interaction with the extra oil and batter. Eight. Serve.

Berry filling

Ingredients

Frozen cherries

10 ouncesFrozen

blueberries – 8 ouncesApple juice – 1 cup Stevia– 1/8 tsp.

Arrowroot powder – 1 tbsp. Water – ¼ cup

Method

1. In a pot, deliver the squeezed apple, blueberries, cherries, and stevia to a bubble over medium heat.

2. Lower the hotness and stew till the herbal merchandise are touchy, round 10 mins.

3. Add arrowroot powder in a bowl, pour the water and mix nicely.

four. Raise hotness to excessive and upload the arrowroot mixture to the dish. Cook and blend for 1 moment, or until the mixture thickens and turns into smooth.

five. Allow the sauce to chill in advance than serving.

Cinnamon Coffee Cake

Ingredients

Cake

Blanched almond flour – 2 ½ cups (no longer almond meal) Celtic sea salt

– ¼ tsp.

Baking soda – ½ tsp. Coconut oil– ¼ cup Honey– ½ cup

Eggs – three massive

Topping

Coconut oil

– ¼ cup, melted Coconut sugar – ¼ cup
Ground cinnamon– 2 tbsp. Sliced almonds – ½
cup

Method

1. With coconut oil, oil a 9-inch spherical cake
subject and afterward dust with almond flour.

2. In a food processor, be part of baking pop,
salt, and almond flour. Three. Pulse within the
eggs, honey, and coconut oil. Four. Spread the
hitter into the pre-arranged baking dish. 5. To
make the garnish: In a touch bowl,
consolidate reduce

almonds, cinnamon, coconut sugar, and
coconut oil.

6. Sprinkle besting over cake batter.

7. Bake for 25 to 35 mins at 350F.

eight. Cool and serve.

Almond Flour Pancakes

Eggs – three large Water – 1 tbsp.

Vanilla extract – 1 tbsp.

Agave nectar or honey– 2 tbsp. Blanched almond flour – 1 ½ cups Celtic sea salt– ¼ tsp.

Baking soda – ¼ tsp.

Coconut oil or grapeseed oil for baking

Method

1. Whisk collectively the eggs, agave, water, and vanilla in a large bowl. 2. Add salt, almond flour, and baking pop and mix properly. Three. In a skillet, warmth oil over medium warmness.

four. For every hotcake, scoop 1 storing tbsp. Participant into the

skillet.

5. Cook till bubbles shape on top, then, at that issue, flip and prepare dinner the opportunity thing.

6. Remove from field and be aware on a plate.

7. Repeat with the extra hitter and serve.

Main

Meals

Lime

Salmon

Salmon – 1 lb. Reduce into four fillets Olive oil – 1 to 2 tbsp.

Limes – 2, sliced in 1/2 Celtic sea salt– 1 tsp.

Chipotle powder – 1 tsp.

Method

1. Preheat the broiler to 500F.

2. Rinse the salmon, wipe off and placed on a metal baking sheet. Three. Rub every filet with olive oil.

four. From one-half of lime, press the juice onto every fillet. Five. Sprinkle filets with chipotle and salt. Then, at that point, on

pinnacle of every filet, vicinity a half of lime.
6. Lower broiler temperature to 275F.

7. Place salmon inside the range and cook dinner for 8 to 12 mins. Time is based totally completely upon the way you need your fish.

Rosemary Apple Chicken

Chicken – 1 entire (2 to 3 pounds) Grapeseed oil or olive oil– ¼ cup Balsamic vinegar – 1/3 cup

Celtic sea salt – 1 tbsp. Apples – 4, cored and sliced Rosemary– 4 sprigs

Method

1. Rinse the hen, wipe off and mounted a baking dish (9 x thirteen inch).

2. Drizzle with vinegar, oil and sprinkle with salt.

three. Arrange the apples in the course of the hen inside the baking dish.

four. Place the branches of rosemary beneath the hen.

five. Bake at 350F till seared outwardly, round ninety mins.

6. Serve.

Meatballs

Ground beef – 1 pound Egg– 1 massive

Shallot – 1, minced Tomato paste– 2 tbsp. Dijon mustard– 2 tbsp. Coconut flour – 1 tbsp. Celtic sea salt– ½ tsp.

Ground black pepper – ½ tsp. Baking soda– ¼ tsp.

Method

1. In a big bowl, be part of egg, shallot, and floor beef.

2. Mix within the coconut flour, mustard, tomato glue, salt, pepper and baking soda.

3. Use a ¼-cup scoop to make meatballs.

four. Line a baking sheet with fabric paper and spot the meatballs. Five. Bake at 350F until a meat thermometer peruses 175F, round 25 minutes.

6. Serve with spaghetti squash noodles.

Mac and Cheese Casserole

Organic grass fed ground pork – 1 lb. Spaghetti squash noodles – 4 cups Heavy cream – ½ cup Eggs – four big

Smoked paprika– 1 tbsp. Celtic sea

salt– 1 tsp.

Ground black pepper – 1 tsp.

Freshly grated parmesan cheese– ½ cup Freshly grated cheddar cheese– 2 cups

Method

1. Cook hamburger till brown in a cast-iron skillet.

2. Remove the hamburger from the hotness. Set aside.

3. Whisk eggs and weighty cream till clean in a bowl.

4. Add smoked paprika and season with salt and pepper.

5. Stir in 1-cup cheddar, parmesan and spaghetti squash. 6. Stir in ground beef.

7. Transfer aggregate decrease lower back to the skillet. Eight. Top with the leftover cheddar.

nine. Bake at 350F for 40 to 50 minutes, or until growing round the edges.

10. Cool 15 minutes and serve.

Spaghetti Squash Noodles

Ingredients

Spaghetti squash– 1 medium, approximately 3 pounds

Method

1. Line a baking sheet with material paper and be conscious entire spaghetti squash.

2. Poke the squash times with a fork.

three. Bake at 350F for 60 to eighty mins.

4. Cool the squash for 30 minutes.

5. Cut squash open with a blade and scoop out the seeds.

6. Scrape the discern out of the squash into wiry noodles.

7. Serve.

Beef Brisket

Brisket – 1 ½ kilos Chicken inventory

– three cups Onion – 1 big, chopped

Garlic– eight cloves, peeled and sliced Mushrooms– 8 oz., sliced Carrots– 8, sliced ½-inch thick Garlic powder – 1 tbsp. Onion powder – 1 tbsp. Celtic sea

salt– ½ tsp.

Method

1. In a slow cooker, location the carrots, mushrooms, garlic, onion, and stock.

2. Sprinkle with onion powder, garlic powder, and salt.

3. Place the beef inside the center.

four. Turn simmering pot on low and put together dinner dinner for 6 to 8 hours.

five. Serve.

Chicken with Cauliflower and Olives

Boneless, skinless chicken breast − 1 pound Fresh thyme sprigs − 1 bunch

Cauliflower − 1 head, reduce into florets Shallot − 1, finely chopped

Olive oil− three tbsp. Celtic sea salt−

½ tsp.

Ground black pepper − 1 tsp. Zest of 1 lemon

Fresh lemon juice − ¼ cup Kalamata olives

− 1 cup, pitted Garlic− 5 cloves, thinly sliced

Method

1. Rinse the fowl bosoms and wipe off with a paper towel. 2. In the lower part of a 7 x

eleven-inch baking dish, unfold thyme springs evenly.

three. Then spot bird and upload cauliflower florets around the chook. Four. In a bowl, be a part of olives, salt, garlic, pepper, olive oil, shallot, lemon zing, and juice.

5. Pour aggregate over the cauliflower and chicken.

6. Keep inside the fridge in a unmarried day.

7. Bake at 400F until cauliflower can be very lots seared, and hen is cooked via, round 45 to fifty five minutes.

eight. Serve.

Desserts

Paleo Vanilla Cupcakes

Coconut flour – ¼ cup Celtic sea salt– 1/eight tsp. Baking soda– 1/eight tsp. Eggs – three large

Palm shortening– ¼ cup Honey– 2 tbsp.

Vanilla extract – 1 tbsp.

Method

1. Combine the coconut flour, baking pop, and salt in a meals processor.

2. Pulse within the honey, shortening, eggs, and vanilla.

three. Line a cupcake area with paper liners and cut up the hitter among every.

four. Bake at 350F for 20 to 24 mins.

five. Cool for 1 hour.

6. Frost with Paleo chocolate frosting.

Chapter 4: Basic Cross Training Terms

If you are not a organized waft teach, here are a few terms and sports sports that need to be clarified preceding to getting started out:

For Time-This implies you could do the workout, gadgets or reps in the fastest time you're capable of do. Then, at that factor, located out an objective of beating that element the following time you do the equal exercise.

AMRAP-This manner "As Many Reps/Rounds As Possible".

Double beneath-While going for walks out with rope, the rope need to cross beneath your toes times in a unmarried bounce. As such, leap rope revolutions in a single jump.

Jumping pull-ups - This is a kind of helped pull-united stateswhere you hop off the ground on the equal time as doing the draw up and arriving at your jaw over the draw up bar

Knees to elbows-While dangling from a draw up bar with constant arms, use your muscular power to check your sanity up inside the air and call them on your elbows.

Pull-ups – Cross getting prepared pull americadislike normal pressure ups. You are authorized to utilize your pressure to swing to get your jawline over the bar. They are otherwise referred to as kipping pull ups.

Thrusters-An engine resembles an overhead press with the hand weight, other than you furthermore need to move right down in the squat. The energy from the squat will let you with getting the load over your head.

Kettlebell swings-You possibly comprehend what an iron weight swing is, but in extensively teaching, you need to try to convey the transportable weight over your head with steady arms.

Burpees-When you do a burpee, you need to get down, so your chest contacts the floor. It isn't needed to do a push-as plenty as stand up; you can utilize your strain. At the issue at the same time as you stand up, you need to hop off the ground collectively at the side of your hands over your head.

Wall ball tosses Using a weighted workout ball or remedy ball, cross down in a squat and detonate up at the same time as hurling the ball excessive on a divider. Get the ball, pass down in a squat over again and repeat.

Sumo deadlift excessive-pulls This is a sumo deadlift joined with an upstanding column. At the high-quality detail of the deadlift, use your electricity carry the bar up to bear top.

Push press-This is an overhead press with a loose weight, however you are authorized to make use of your legs and strain to get the bar over your head.

Floor wipers- While lying on your decrease once more, increase your ft vertically in the air and (toes together) swing them to the left till you touch the floor, then supply them again up after which over to the right and decrease again and so on. Squat smooth-It is essentially a clean with a the the front squat proper in a while.

Snatch-In one motion, deliver the hand weight starting from the earliest degree, as a protracted way as possible over your head with hands extended.

Following are a couple of instances of Cross Training WODs: 1. 20 Pull-ups, 30 Push-ups, 40 Sit-americaand 50 Squats (Repeat 5 times)

While pull-ups, push-ups, and sit down-u.S.Are apparent for a superb many people, doing a squat calls for the best shape to stay a ways from damage.

For amateurs, start doing squats with out a weight till you have got the right shape. To do the precise squat, function the toes at shoulder width and reduce the body all of the way right down to a squat characteristic.

Do 50 squats every set for a sum of 5 repetitions.

2. Five Handstand Push-ups, 10 1-Legged Squats, and 15 Pull-americaDo "However many Rounds As is probably allowed" rapidly (in any other case known as AMRAP).

To play out a handstand move up start through stooping down at the ground, with the person's lower lower returned confronting a chair.

Place the ft on top of the seat and with the fingers broadened, repair the legs so the hips are introduced up in a V feature. Twist the elbows and reduce head to the ground in a push-up characteristic. Broaden your arms surely returning and rehash five times.

To do 1-legged squats, start with almost no weight and stay on one leg. With the opposite leg raised, deliver down the leg inside the direction of the floor on the identical time as retaining the again directly.

three. 1 Mile Run, three hundred Bodyweight Squats, hundred-Push-ups, a hundred Pull-ups

To do a bodyweight squat, live with the legs shoulder width separated. With the arms at once out in advance than the shoulders, twist the knees and in shape ahead on the midsection on the identical time as maintaining the again immediately.

Benefits of Strength Training

Whether you choice to get more wholesome, located on weight, in addition make bigger your wellbeing, similarly increase your exhibition in a selected game, or clearly experience better and further completely happy, you could accomplish your targets with the boom of harmony making prepared for your life-style.

Aerobic exercise is vital, however to accomplish the amazing results, you need to be part of cardiovascular exercise with strength schooling.

The blessings are in no manner-ending, they encompass:

Decreasing muscle in preference to fats . As you educate, your digestion accelerates and consumes more noteworthy stages of power 24 hours constant with day. Strength making organized can help with switching everyday decreases for your digestion that takes location throughout the time of 30.

Incr eased muscle, bone, tendon and ligament electricity, prompting an lousy lot lots less wounds and plenty a great deal much less scientific troubles in later life, i.E., forestalling osteoporosis.

Improving your stance – As you gain electricity and research exquisite shape, your stance will decorate, and you could stand at once and assured.

Increasing your strength – Greater endurance, adaptability and electricity will offer you with extra power and delight in all elements of your existence.

Chapter 5: Constructing a Fitness Program

When you start a bit out time table, be smooth near what you choice to perform and description a realistic purpose that you may point for.

This motive can be expected in weight, inches, fats price, planned accomplishments, preferred clothing, pulse or cholesterol levels...... Something works for you as an individual.

Once you've got installation a drawn out reason, separate this proper right into a improvement of quick movement dreams.

Think about the time you're inclined and geared up to make available to perform the ones goals, end what season of day will best fit your needs and what weather you need to prepare in.

Choose a technique for making organized that incorporates your person; do you spur yourself and like to prepare on my own?

Do you need the assist and luxury of others and may need to check a preparation associate or person teacher?

Remember, to get the extraordinary outcomes; you want to recognize what you're doing.

Once you recognize what you are focusing on and the manner you could fuse the schooling, you need to make every meeting as treasured as you can.

Take estimations/photos in advance than you start so you can outline your advancement. Keep a diary to file your reps, hundreds, applications, and development.

Try to finish a power educational assembly every next day, ensuring you replacement muscle gatherings and supply a few component like 48 hours rest to every unique place.

Each electricity assembly want to endure from 1/2-hour to an hour in length.

B egin your meetings with compound sports (such as more than one muscle bunch, i.E., Squats, Rows, Bench Press) and later on hold directly to separation works out (using in reality one muscle bunch, i.E., Bicep twists) this will will assist you to capitalize in your muscles with out starting to be too exhausted early on.

Construct the quantity of redundancies and lays out to fit your dreams: For electricity (electricity), 2-6 reiterations, relaxation among sets so long as 2 mins. For hypertrophy (period) 8-12 redundancies, relaxation amongst gadgets so long as 2 minutes. For perseverance, 20-forty redundancies, rest amongst units 30 seconds.

Complete 3 arrangements of each hobby , that means to exhaustion your muscle companies inside the ultimate couple of reps of the second one and 1/3 set. If you are without problem completing all 3 sets (with extremely good form), then waft as plenty as a better weight. Assuming you are trying to finish a set, drop down a weight level.

Follow all protection suggestions; warming up, stretching, cooling down, hydration, vitamins, and lots of others. All are critical on your results and your safety.

Practise your structure, be slow and controlled, watch your self in a mirror, request to be studied, it's miles pivotal your muscle tissues take in extraordinary sports from the start.

To assure your muscle tissue get the pride they need to make bigger, increment your obstruction thru the use of round 10% every three to 4 weeks.

Alter your bodily sports at everyday c programming language s, no matter whether or no longer or no longer it's miles in reality the request to your sports activities activities, this can stop your muscle mass adjusting in your everyday.

Measuring Success

Coming up next are the technique for estimating your very non-public accomplishment in Cross Training;

Medical Results

The health practitioner can will permit you to apprehend your ldl cholesterol level, blood strain, heart charge, and masses of others. These are all numbers that may be monitored for development inside the course of your fitness software and will offer a exceptional incentive for trade as you assist enhance the satisfactory or even length of your existence.

Weight on the size

Be careful whilst passing judgment on development with the useful resource of the usage of weight by myself, variances are normal and deceiving. You need to definitely take a perusing one time each week, at that very hour of the day. Recollect as you get in shape in fat, you're additionally acquiring muscle weight, and your state-of-the-art scales don't apprehend the difference.

Clothing

If your goal is weight reduction, a component of apparel which you need to put on may be a sturdy percentage of development. Giving or re-measuring garb that is too massive will assist with forestalling you getting lower decrease lower back to antique lousy behavior.

Abilities

If you can run further in a specific time, increase a extra distinguished weight, accomplish extra reps, stretch further, hop better, score extra tries, play at the side of your kids longer - some thing is essential to you, employ that as a marker for achievement.

four Safe Training Strategies

Before starting a training software, it is prescribed to talk approximately your preparations with a medical care talented, specifically assuming you haven't practiced for a couple of years, are extra than 35 years of age, overweight or experiencing a health state of affairs.

Before training continuously stretch out and warmth up your muscular tissues. An suitable heat-up will hoist the heart beat and increment blood waft to the functioning muscle mass which bring about lots much less threat of harm, similarly advanced execution and dwindled muscle stiffness.

Make fine you stretch the muscles so one may be centered on at some stage in exercise. A recommended heat-up is probably slight on foot or bypass with some frame weight bodily sports which encompass push united statescombined with a few static stretches. An choice heat-up is to play out the sports activities that you will bear in mind to your exercise but just to raise 25-1/2 of of the weight.

1. Maintain proper stance and approach

2. Do now not bend or curve your again. Keep your frame even, settle your center, manage

each development, middle round the problem you are doing and which muscle tissue are in use.

3. NEVER CONTINUE TRAINING IF YOU FEEL PAIN

4. Don't overlook to respire

Take robust, complete breaths. Inhale out for the duration of strive (the difficult aspect of the interest) and take in at the move decrease again (the smooth issue). Breathing out through your enamel with a murmuring sound can assist on the same time as you're engaged, and your muscle companies are gotten smaller and strolling tough.

five. Stay hydrated in the end of your exercising

Have a jug of water nearby; drink like clockwork, your exhibition will endure at the off hazard that you are dehydrated.

6. After your work out, calm down

A cool down is a regular however normal decline inside the interest alongside extending and rehydration. Around five-10 minutes of mild energetic motion will

assist to keep blood from pooling in fringe enlarged veins and abatement the opportunity of blacking out or muscle squeezing while moreover helping with retaining apart any lactic corrosive that might anyways be to be had in your muscle agencies.

7. Rest and Recovery

Resting amongst adjusts is critical to get higher your muscle tissues restrict. Try not to make it too short time frame or your muscle organizations obtained't have efficaciously recuperated and you'll not be capable of perform similarly to is probably expected, but don't stand by means of the usage of the usage of excessively long or your pulse will lessen, and you may lose middle. Between 60-ninety seconds is a sincere diploma of recovery time. Utilize an possibility to have a beverage, stretch or truely inhale profound. Resting among instructional courses is important; your muscle tissues are growing at some degree in the healing time. Don't over prepare, as your muscle mass received't have had the opportunity to repair themselves. Substitute muscle gatherings, take rest days wherein you in fact do no education via any technique and get an entire lot of fee sleep.

eight. Follow splendid healthy conduct

It is pivotal for development and restoration which you provide your body ok fuel to work and a tremendous equilibrium of protein, fiber, starches, and fats to live stable and achieve your fitness objectives. Eat constantly and all subjects considered, avoid dealt with food, soaked fat, and some of alcohol.

9. Stay healthful

An greater safety tip respects cleanliness; severa microscopic organisms and infections thrive in a rec middle weather (even your own home exercising middle), usually use your towel, wash your wraps, wipe down the sack with a sanitizer splash and easy up previous to ingesting, presence of mind can stop infection.

Reasons to Stretch

Correct extending is valuable for increasing adaptability and as a quit result will assist with every damage counteraction and harm treatment.

If you supply a muscle or ligament m ore distinguished scope of motion while it's miles uninvolved, it's far going to be dubious to come across tears at the equal time as finished actively.

Combining a warm up and growing before exercising will organized the muscle tissues

for movement and lessening the threat of damage. As the nerves to muscle pathways are prepared, co-appointment will beautify, and you can experience a decline in muscle anxiety.

Chapter 6: Stretching Suggestions

NECK EXTENSION

1. Stand tall, shoulders once more and down; center exchanged on.

2. Gently tip your head back until your eyes are admiring the sky, you want to sense the stretch beneath your chin.

three. Hold this situation for five-10 seconds.

4. Return to the midline function before repeating.

CHIN GLIDE (Neck Extensors)

1. Stand tall, shoulders again and down; center exchanged on. 2. Slowly skim your jaw beforehand (like a chicken) and in a while withdraw your jaw and drop your jawline down closer to your chest.

three. Hold every characteristic for 5-10 seconds.

four. Return to the midline function previous to rehashing. NECK ROTATION (Neck Rotators)

1. Stand tall, shoulders again and down; middle exchanged on.

2. Gently flip head apart, so your jawline comes round, and you may check out your shoulder. You have to fondle the stretch the aspect of your neck you have got have been given disregarded from.

three. Hold this case for five-10 seconds.

4. Return to the midline characteristic previous to rehashing. HORIZONTAL NECK FLEXION

1. Stand tall, shoulders decrease decrease again and down; middle exchanged on.

2. Gently twist your head apart, so your ear attracts in the direction of your shoulder

three. Hold this case for five-10 seconds.

four. Return to midline function previous to rehashing on the alternative component.

5. To delicately construct energy you could placed your give up your head to help with supplying to it fairly closer to your shoulder

TRICEP STRETCH (Triceps Brachii)

1. Place one palm stage on your pinnacle decrease again, in conjunction with your elbow pointing in the direction of the ceiling.

2. Use your other hand to pull the elbow in closer to your head gently. Three. Hold this situation for 20-forty seconds.

Benefits of Using Dumbbells

There are such limitless ways of strolling out, however the maximum perfect way is the most effective that is simplest to fuse into your manner of existence and which you could apprehend whilst engaging in remarkable effects.

For those motives and severa others, loose weights are high-quality for all ranges of well-being and some thing your athletic goals can be.

Dumbbells are less high priced and correctly available .

Dumbbells don't want masses of room to be used.

Dumbbells are portable.

Dumbbells can be executed in a massive quantity of sports.

The outcomes completed the usage of hand weights are often higher compared to the ones accomplished on rec center machines.

Using hand weights in addition develops general and coordination.

Dumbbell practices aren't tough to have a have a look at and don't forget. HAND WEIGHT SAFETY

Follow all the fitness making equipped strategies.

Exercise in a degree clean location liberated from interruptions .Ensure you're following proper form constantlyProgress step by step and securely, start each new exercise with a mild weight.

Store your loose weights securely in a rack among employments.

Whenever plausible make use of a Spotter:

A spotter is any character who's available that will help you assuming that you lose your surplus or

come to be too exhausted to even maintain in thoughts completing an interest all by myself securely. They need to recognize about their security when supporting you and feature themselves wherein they received't thwart your trends, but in which they'll abruptly flow to help you if important. Their hands want to be close to your wrists or beneath the loose weights due to overhead lifts.

Equipments Option

SPRING LOADED ECONOMY DUMBBELLS

A plenty less luxurious choice to the movable spinlock hand weights. Regularly empty, those handles may not maintain comparable capacities of weight. Be that as it may, they can be a amazing choice for amateurs, and the spring collars remember speedy weight adjustments.

ADJUSTABLE INTERLOCKING DUMBBELLS

Instead of screwing plates onto a deal with, you lock on greater weight regions as needed to a focal middle weight block. This is an incredibly minimized association and takes into attention rapid modifications in weight.

A FID BENCH (FLAT/INCLINE/DECLINE)

A very plenty deliberate seat permits you to play out an great scope of sports. When related to the seat in a stage feature, you can set up your toes on the floor and feature place to deliver your elbows/hands/masses beneath the quantity of your frame. Slight changes inside the factors of slope and rot mean you could intention particular muscle businesses even as preserving up with tremendous shape on a regular creation. Pick a strong metallic seat with an all spherical cushioned top and easy, steady, bendy elements.

A TOWEL AND WATER BOTTLE

A towel is incredible for placing down over your seat for introduced cleanliness. A towel is likewise had to clean off sweat to hold your draw close secure on the hardware. Keep a jug of water near continually so that you can re-hydrate in your rest durations.

AN EXERCISE/FIT BALL

A modest embellishment that might assist outcomes, reinforcing your middle and with mission higher

similarly developing your equilibrium. Numerous kinds of sports activities can be improved thru sitting or mendacity on an hobby ball. Buy a period that suits your peak

Legs

It is important to have a sturdy base to growth on for a legitimate frame, and that suggests sturdy legs.

Work with moderate masses on the same time as finishing leg works out, your frame weight will offer the superb majority of the competition required.

To make a proportioned frame and all round created legs, make sure to exercising the the the front (Quadriceps) and all over again (Hamstring) muscle tissues of the thigh, simply because the Calves.

Stretch properly previous to training your legs and heat up via mild exercising or cardio to guarantee you accomplish your great effects in the course of your exercising and keep away from damage.

Hamstrings: Biceps Femoris, Semitendinosus, and Semimembranosus

PILE SQUAT (Quadriceps, Hamstrings, GluteusMaximus, ErectorSpinae)

1. Stand ft shoulder-width separated, knees marginally bowed. Center grew to come to be on, instantly decrease lower back, center inside the front.

2. Hold a solitary loose weight, getting a address in the path of 1 aspect from above with palms, so it is placing before you on immediately fingers.

three. Hinge at your hips and drop right away down, staying your backside out like plunking down. Keep your chest up and don't allow your knees to transport out earlier than your toes. Drop all over again into your hips to the extent you're succesful, ideally till your pinnacle legs are similar to the ground. Four. Pause in quick on the lower part of the squat and afterward breathe out as you force down via your impact factors and push your hips in advance to get over again to status.

DUMBBELL THRUSTER (Quadriceps, Glutes, Deltoids, Triceps) 1. Stand with your ft shoulder-width separated, knees marginally twisted, middle have become on, Focus inside the front.

2. Hold a free weight in each hand and lift them to a beginning state of affairs over every shoulder. Palms confronting together

3. Hinge at your hips and drop right away down, staying your rump out like plunking down. Drop all over again into your hips to the quantity you're capable, in a in truth ideal worldwide until your pinnacle legs are similar to the floor.

four. Pause on the decrease a part of the squat and in a while breathe out as you stress down through your heels and push your hips ahead to get to repute.

5. As you rise over again to reputation, press the two hand weights flawlessly overhead till your fingers are right now, but not locked out.

Chest

The chest is the gap of the frame the diverse neck and the center. The key muscle companies that make up the chest location are PECTORALIS MAJOR and PECTORALIS MINOR.

The chest place includes likely the most important muscle bunches within the better frame.

When you workout your chest, your shoulders and arms are likewise concerned. So a chest workout can likewise pass about as a get ready for those muscle mass.

You can increase large masses using your chest muscle organizations, however need to constantly assure you improvement step by step and employ the excellent shape to save you damage on your chest and shoulders.

Include some warm temperature up sets in your exercising and allow some days rest after a weighty chest workout to broaden development and restore.

BENCH PRESS (PectoralisMajor, Triceps, AnteriorDeltoid) 1. On a seat, lie degree in your again, so your head is upheld. Twist your knees and each plant your ft on the ground, or spot them on the end of the seat, certainly aside.

2. If you don't have a spotter to assist you with stepping into and out of function, increase the loose weights onto your thighs, in any case and in a while roll lower decrease back even as elevating the hand weights to in reality beneath your armpits.

3. Switch your center on, and with a free weight held in each hand (palms inside the route of your ft), expand your arms up until they are almost proper now and the hand weights are held degree over your shoulders.

4. Keep your back in contact with the seat constantly. Bring down the hand weights in a lethargic controlled manner, cutting down each unfastened weight to the outdoor facets of your chest.

five. Before respiratory out prevent at the identical time as raising the loose weights step by step again to the start function.

PULLOVER (PectoralisMajor, PectoralisMinor, LatissimusDorsi

)

1. On a seat, lie degree in your lower back, so your head is upheld. Twist your knees and both plant your feet on the ground, or spot them at the give up of the seat, certainly aside.

2. Hold one loose weight among palms, fingers confronting the roof. Fix your fingers and hold the loose weight over your mid-chest.

three. Keeping your again in touch with the seat continuously, bring down the hand weight in the again of your head the amount that you may obtain.

4. Pause in short, preceding to taking the hand weight grade by grade again to the start

characteristic. Keep up with immediately hands and nonstop manipulate.

Back

The once more is the region from the very best component of the posterior to the rear of the neck and shoulders.

Muscles inside the lower again are engaged with the improvement of the neck and bears and the protected development and assure of the spine. The pinnacle lower back gives basically underlying assist on the same time as the lower yet again has more noteworthy adaptability and motion.

Back torment through muscle strain is as a substitute everyday; always stretch and warm up, in no manner over-stress and STOP IMMEDIATELY IF YOU EXPERIENCE PAIN.

If you have got skilled once more torment, constantly propose a scientific professional preceding to starting each exclusive well-being regime.

DEADLIFT (ErectorSpinae, GluteusMaximus, Hamstrings) 1. Stand feet hip width separated with a slight curve in your knees. Center exchanged on.

2. Keep right now fingers together with your arms searching into your body due to the fact the loose weight is to your palms.

three. Hinge forward from the hips and as you deliver down your chest vicinity (which remains in unbiased arrangement); permit your knees to curve a bit. Keep your arms right now and close to your legs subsequently of the exercise.

4. Go as little as your adaptability permits. Keep your pay interest descending to try not to strain your neck.

five. Pause in short at the decrease a part of the motion, preceding to breathing out even as pushing thru your heels to getting another time to status.

SEATED BENT OVER FLY (MiddleTrapezius, Rhomboids, PosteriorDeltoids)

1. Sit at the constrained finish of a seat and pivot ahead from your middle, so you are twisted right over.

2. The loose weight need to be held in every deliver over thru your lower legs, hands confronting internal. Switch your middle on, center across the ground.

three. In a torpid controlled improvement, enhance the hand weights up, maintaining your hands almost instantly until they come on the volume of your shoulders. Breathe out and press your shoulder bones collectively as you raise your hands.

4. Pause in short, preceding to bringing the hand weight often right right all the way down to the begin function. Try not to move your legs or middle throughout the exercising.

Shoulders

The muscular tissues and joints that make the shoulder permit improvement through an first-rate scope of feelings. This versatility implies the shoulder is moreover temperamental, willing to numerous wounds and should all the time be dealt with with care.

Use proper form in the course of all activities and warmth up your muscle corporations before your exercise.

BENT OVER FLY (Trapezius, Rhomboids, PosteriorDeltoid) 1. Stand proper away and in some time pivot ahead specifically at your hips and stick your backside decrease again a hint.

2. Hold a loose weight in every hand, palm confronting each other and hands nearly immediately and according collectively in conjunction with your legs. Switch your center on.

three. Keeping your wrists without delay, press your shoulder bones down and collectively as you beautify every your hands up and outward until they may be just like the floor.

4. Pause in brief at the very satisfactory factor of the movement preceding to bringing the hand weights progressively right down to the start feature.

5. To gather the stress of this hobby, pivot in advance undeniably, the most excessive being the thing at which your center is similar to the ground.

BENT OVER DELTOID PRESS (Trapezius, Posterior&LateralDeltoids) 1. Stand right away on the side of your feet constant shoulder width separated. Pivot beforehand from your hips and stick your backside lower once more a bit.

2. The loose weight need to be held in each hand, palm confronting every different, hands twisted ninety ranges on the elbow and top palms in accordance collectively along with your shoulders. Switch your center on.

Chapter 7: Suggestions for Exercise

BARBELL SHRUG (UpperTrapezius, LevatorScapulae)

1. Stand along with your toes round shoulder-width separated, transfer your middle on, middle within the front.

2. With a immediately again and without a doubt bowed knees, cope with a unfastened weight with an overhand hold highly extra terrific than shoulder-width separated and return to status.

three. With a solid again and middle, keep your fingers truely proper away as you shrug your shoulders right now up toward your ears. Try not to pivot your shoulders in contrary or use your palms to boost the bar.

four. Pause for a couple of moments preceding to bringing your shoulders proper right down to the beginning situation in a lethargic managed manner.

5. A variety is to raise the free weight behind you lower back, maintain close together

collectively together with your arms confronting in contrary. Follow a comparable shape as above, maintaining your fingers right away and raising your shoulders directly as plenty as the furthest amount that you can float.

UPRIGHT ROW (Deltoids, UpperTrapezius)

1. Stand collectively along with your feet round shoulder-width separated, transfer your middle on, center within the the front

2. With a right away another time and certainly bowed knees, cope with a unfastened weight with an overhand draw close particularly more notable than shoulder-width aside.

three. With at once fingers, stand upstanding bringing the bar up to install your thighs. This is the start function.

4. With locked wrists and a sturdy decrease lower back and middle, breathe out as you frequently pull the hand weight up in your focal chest. (To stay a ways from

shoulder strain, don't increase the bar any better) As you boom gift expectancies, preserve it near your body and assure your elbows are up higher all the time than your wrists.

five. Pause for multiple moments previous to bringing the bar all the way down to the beginning situation in a lethargic managed way.

INCLINE BENCH PRESS (UpperPectorals, Triceps, AnteriorDeltoids)

1. Adjust a seat to a degree of spherical 30 ranges incline.

2. Lie down to your lower returned on a seat together collectively with your lower again level and your feet constant hip-width separated on the ground. The bar ought to be located over your head.

3. Grasp the bar with an overhand preserve mainly more significant than shoulder-width aside.

4. Switch your center on and remove the bar from the rack and maintain it with at once palms at once over your mid-chest. Guarantee your shoulders are decrease again and your chest is up.

five. Slowly in addition the bar down until your better fingers are nearly similar to the ground. Try not to permit the bar to contact your chest.

6. Pause for a couple of moments prior to breathing out and pushing the bar often vertically till your hands are instantly yet again.

BENCH PRESS (PectoralisMajor, AnteriorDeltoid, Triceps) 1. Lie down to your again on a seat together with your head upheld, lower once more stage and your feet regular hip-width separated on the floor or upon a robust platform.

2. Clasp the band with an overhand deal with extremely greater huge than shoulder-width aside.

three. Switch your middle on, dispose of the bar from the rack and keep it with at once hands immediately over your mid-chest. Guarantee your shoulders are again and your chest is up.

four. Slowly in addition the bar down till your higher fingers are similar to the floor. Try not to permit the bar to touch your chest.

five. Pause for multiple moments preceding to respiration out and pushing the bar step by step vertically till your hands are straight away again.Bench press practices using a stage seat, attention on the focal filaments of the Pectoralis Major. Utilizing a decay seat will positioned more accentuation at the decrease strands of Pectoralis Major. Utilizing a grade seat will placed greater accentuation at the pinnacle strands of Pectoralis Major.

SIT-UP AND PRESS (RectusAbdominus, PectoralisMajor, Deltoids, Triceps)

1. Lie all the manner down to your once more on a degree or slope seat at the side of your head supported and your yet again flat.

2. Ensure your feet are degree on the floor, or your lower legs are gotten to the lower leg pads.

three. Grasp the hand weight with an overhand keep shoulder-width separated and rest the bar softly in your higher chest.

4. Switch your center on.

5. Raise yourself up thru getting your abs. Breathe out as you play out a managed sit down down-up on the same time as at the identical time squeezing the free weight as masses as an overhead position.

6. Breathe in as you circulate frequently all of the way right down to the seat while at the equal time returning the hand weight to your chest.

Chapter 8: Benchmark the Girls

'The Girls' are benchmark carrying activities are purported to gauge the enhancements in your exhibition, they will be to be finished irregularly.

The "Young ladies" is basically a gaggle of locating out sports activities sports finished without a big

utilization of hardware this is weighty. These, as the selection proposes, are very suitable for girls, but are the primary Cross Training benchmark practices given to guys and ladies alike.

But those WODs are very powerful and checking out, and some instances definitely debilitating, and all Cross Training opposition wanting to get prepared to shape want to do that. These Girls consume power and acquire muscle like no exquisite, and they're able to draw you nearer on your superb body in little or no time.

Angie

Complete the

interest one hundred squats

one hundred sit down-ups

one hundred push-ups

100 pressure ups

Barbara

five rounds for

time 50

squats

40 take a seat-ups

30 push-ups

20 draw ups

Cindy

Do massive numbers of these

quickly of: 6 draw ups

10 push-ups

15 squats

Grace

30 reps for time

Clean and jerk

135lbs

Helen

3 rounds for time

4 hundred-meter run

1.Five pood iron weight swing x

21 Pullups 12 reps

Isabel

30 reps for time

Snatch a hundred thirty five kilos

Jackie

For time

1000 meter line

Thruster 45lbs – 50 reps

Pullups – 30 reps

Karen

For time

Wall-ball – 100 fifty pix

Linda (furthermore called 'three

bars of death') Deadlift 1.Five

BW

Bench 1x BW

Clean ¾ BW

Annie

50-forty-30-20-10 rep adjusts for time Reps
of:

Doubleunders

Sit-ups

Lynne

five rounds for optimum reps (no longer timed)

Bodyweight seat press (assuming you weigh 170lbs, you can seat 170lbs) Pull-ups

Nicole

As many rounds as feasible in a brief

time of: Run 400m

Max rep pull-ups

Chapter 9: How to Prevent Injury

The hazard of Cross Training, although, aren't clearly the physical video video games but extra so credited to helpless way and a lack of oversight that is taking a constantly growing fee for shoulders, however hips, knees and typically the decrease back.

Cross Training isn't new the usage of any and all way. Much in reality so it modified into stopped via many training divisions again within the 1990's because of the damage toll a few of the men... Also those were guys searching extraordinary! Picture such centered energy and appeal sporting activities being completed through the normal Joe and Jill Average?! Is all people surprised that wounds are on the rise?

And Cross Training Trainers themselves are not invulnerable with numerous physiotherapists making prepared the coaches in a way to treat their minor muscle court cases.

Body Leadership Australia physio, Paul Trevethan, likewise concurs that the acute interest and to a excellent amount aggressive residences of the Cross Training device increment the shot at harm. He likewise concedes that wounds are essentially coming from the"decrease degree competitor that is available in and is going gung-ho.".

So Do The Benefits Outweigh The Dangers Of Cross Training? Look, when you endure in thoughts everything, Cross Training is a beautiful method that makes awesome effects. It absolutely isn't a fledgling or possibly transitional level workout software program. It have become meant for our international class powers so that during itself need to offer you with a few thing of view into what is needed to because it ought to be but in addition securely complete this kind of software program program.

The damage risk can appear like excessive, and no character would in all likelihood deny the greater than best frequency charge of mainly shoulder injuries however the terrible talk about Cross Training is way over the pinnacle close to the opinion of many Cross Training on foot shoes like Matt Noonan and Aidan Rich, an Australian Physiotherapy spokesperson.

While Mr. Rich perceived that there was an event of shoulder wounds, the nicely-being and health benefit a ways over-shadowed the negatives. Coach Matt Noonan likewise sees eye to eye that the harm hazard is low insofar as customers have been established the proper gadget and they had been carefully supervised.

Cross Training is a top notch program, however it need to be endeavored with the useful resource of the use of the ones looking tremendous, hoping to settle the rating more out of their health places and apprehend extra noteworthy results. If you are acting at a immoderate modern-day and need a brand new project then in reality circulate for it. In any case, any person who's at fledgling or halfway diploma need to reevaluate their goals and actual capacities previous to attempting Cross Training.

As generally while in the exercise center, fantastic form and running out below manipulate is in fact so large and need to in no way be constrained. The equal is going twofold for Cross Training getting geared up however finished accurately and carried out right, Cross Training will undertaking you need no unique workout software, and I encourage you to have a cross assuming that you are feeling as tons because it.

Again as fashionable, talk together with your huge scientific expert or doctor at some thing component you are going to begin a few distinctive exercising regime! Getting into form and further developing your unity and well-being is exceptional for every person and there isn't any "one length suits all" workout time desk. It's likewise not tied in with beating every other character however alternatively yourself and you that changed into the day past, or closing week or perhaps a 12 months ago! Chapter 21: Some recommendation from Cross Trainers

We can credit score score rating the begin of the Cross Training habitual to Coach Greg Glassman. He has spent numerous years growing and calibrating the specifics of this software program program. He accepts that any health habitual need to set up its followers for any sudden scenario. Without a doubt, this appears to be the inspiration of the Cross making ready recurring. The schooling session regimes mean to set up all who keep on with the program for any real undertaking that an individual might also additionally be called upon to carry out.

Chapter 10: Benefits of Cross-Training

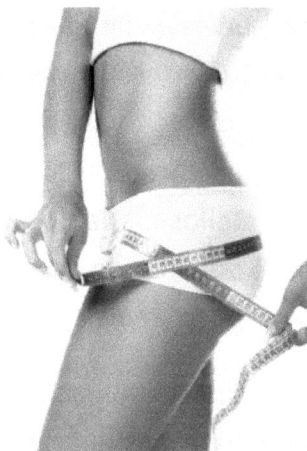

If you have got been doing conventional health packages, carrying sports and gambling sports activities sports as a shape of workout for some time, you have got probably been thinking why they don't placed on you out that without problems any greater. Or while you play a few hoops together together together with your pals for greater than an hour, you're even though top to move? Or likely you've been looking to recognize why you haven't been seeing very many consequences for pretty a while.

It's because of the fact you've been doing the ones sports activities for a long time and your body has had been given used to them. Your frame isn't getting sore anymore, and those sports aren't tiring you very masses anymore. You're muscular, cardiovascular and anxious systems have tailor-made to those sorts of stimulae and your body isn't forced to grow, evolve and adapt anymore.

That is why pass-schooling is one of these outstanding recreations. It might be an entire new revel in in order to do masses of proper to your body.

Conditioning your body through manner of doing an entire lot of carrying sports which preserve changing with each workout is a splendid start. Gradually developing the worload also can be very useful.

Cross-schooling packages will help you lose fats, gain muscle and provide a lift on your aerobic-aerobic potential. Plus, you will gather a brand new set of abilties with all of the new movements within the physical sports activities. Also, if you do the whole thing right, you are not feasible to reason any harm to yourself.

Repetitive wearing activities and applications will bore you out. We as humans, are stimulated via the usage of range and most of really dislike monotony. Cross-schooling, with its wonderful WODs, motivates you to artwork more difficult every day, pushes you to overcome your PR's and enables you keep your enthusiasm for fitness. Cross-education has one-of-a-type bodily activities in-keep for you with the intention to push each a part of your frame to its restrict. Thus making you extra healthy and making you carry out excellently in races or contests. It moreover lets in you to be flexible in making options approximately your schooling wishes and plans.

In gyms, it's usually fine a group of random humans doing exceptional workout workouts. But in pass-education, you are in a network. Although you could regularly compete with others in case you want, on the save you of the day it's no longer about competing with others, but with yourself. In this community, human beings not most effective push themselves, however in addition they enthusiastically root for others.

If you take delivery of as true with you studied you're going to hide your weaknesses, suppose once more. The humans at pass-education make their weaknesses visible so that they have the hazard to improve them and to excel in disciplines which might be their prone factors. And this software program isn't handiest for men as many humans frequently count on. The girls can and do take part too. Young or antique, girl or male, they're all right right here to enhance their lives and so need to you.

Cross-schooling Equipment and What You Need to Know About It

The 'critical' machine list:

Mats: You need to usually have those for protection and luxury allows to hold you from slipping and falling.

The Jump Rope: cheap and splendid aerobic tool.

Weight-lifting bar and plates: desired while doing squats, cleans, jerks, presses, snatches, deadlifts, thrusters and one-of-a-type carrying occasions.

Bumper plates: there are normal weights, however in case you take place to drop them, what is going to arise is you, your weights and the ground can go through.

Rings: you could use the ones for extra motives you could take into account. Just maintain them available and also you'll find an area to maintain them.

Kettlebell: a solid iron or metallic weight used to perform ballistic sports that integrate cardiovascular, energy and flexibility schooling. You can start out with 20 lbs or 35lbs.

Climbing rope: a 20-foot rope will do the trick. What to do with it? Why now not strive putting it on a tree and mountaineering it in case you don't have acces to a community circulate-education 'place'?

Rower: A special machine that simulates the actions of sitting an rowing in a deliver. It is a evry notable shape of cardiovascular workout.

Flat bench: this piece of device is a want in your WODs.

Squat rack: an object of weight schooling tool designed to permit for a free-weight workout using a barbell with out the motion regulations.

Pull Up Bar: you can purchase this however ensure it's far sturdy sufficient to assist your weight. You don't want to move swinging to the clinic.

GHD or Glute Hamstring Devolper: It is good in constructing your lower once more and if used in any other case, it'll end result to excellent ab burning take a seat-ups.

Dumbbells and Dumbbells Rack: make sure you get some of dumbbell weights to compliment your WOD sports from the lightest to the heaviest.

Weight tree: I ought to endorse which you get a weight tree. It will unclutter your floor and provide you with an a whole lot less complex time while converting weights.

Additional topics to keep in mind:

Music –The proper shape of track can help you get thru the difficult WODs.

Electric fan / air conditioner / heater

Gymnast Hand Chalk: gymnast hand chalk can surely help together along side your grip whilst doing the kettlebell WODs.

White Board or Blackboard: To jot down your times.

Stop watch: a useful device to record your timing whilst doing the WODs.

Kettlebells

If you need weightlifting, because of the effective effects on your body, specifically your muscle tissues, mental control and conditioning, similarly to the improve that it offers yourself-self warranty, then you may defenitely experience kettlebell sporting sports activities and workout exercises. Kettlebells are considered to be one of the nice methods to develop your strength, mobility, flexibility and staying power.

A kettlebell seems like a steel ball, typically black, that has a U-fashioned control on its pinnacle which serves as its cope with.You have probably already seen it usually before. It is available in numerous weights, this is painted or embossed on both factor of the kettlebell. But no longer all kettlebells are round. They are used to flex and expand the muscle groups with the resource of retaining and moving it in particular methods. It is held by way of the U-shapped bar with the aid of the palm and utilized by elevating or decreasing it to achieve muscle anxiety in your desired body detail. Kettlebells can usually be offered in sports activities sports stores international and can be presented in bulk with unique grades of weight, occasionally with a kettlebell rack covered.

Although its beginning is quite uncertain, it is been stated through numerous human beings that Kettlebells originated from Ancient Greece. The evidence of that could be a 143-kg kettlebell displayed on the Archeological Museum in Olympia with an inscription written on it that announces, "Bibon heaved up me above the top through the use of one hand". It continued for use in Russia in which it changed into published of their authentic dictionary in 1704 as "Girya", kettlebells, in a while, have become known as what it's far nowadays. Athletes the use of kettlebells as part of their exercise are known as "Gireviks" and the sport wherein kettlebells are used is referred to as the "Girevoy" recreation. Kettlebells were utilized in the earlier years of Russia as a measuring device for grains and different exchangeable gadgets. Athletes again then knowledgeable using kettlebells incorporating them in a unmarried-of-a-kind athletic video video games and activities. According to them, even though kettlebells develop power, and that they do not offer a cumbersome look to the frame.

In 1948, fifty 5 athletes attended the primary kettlebell competition in Russia. "Gireviks" (kettlebell athletes) made use of 3 disciplines in kettlebell competition, the jerk, press, and take preserve of. Later on, one day spherical 1974, it have become an ethnic game in Russia with most effective disciplines left, the jerk and the grab. Alongside like weightlifting, the click was removed from the sport. There were many modifications in kettlebell sports activities activities because of the fact then. Many suggestions have been changed or eliminated. Up till nowadays, kettlebell lifting is considered as a exercising with fantastic sports spread the world over. European Union of Weightball Lifting (later called International Union of Kettlebell Lifting) was created lower back in 1992 wherein the primary European kettlebell championship modified into held.

The kettlebell, as a weightlifting and exercise tool, end up first introduced in American magazines once more inside the past due 20's and in the long run delivered to at the least one-of-a-kind components of the western international locations.

Kettlebell traning is now a distinguished shape of exercise and fitness that is practiced via many human beings in diverse nations, every in eastern and western components of the arena.

Kettlebell lifting has been considered a sports activities sports activities vicinity for the purpose that time whilst considered one of a kind weightlifting strategies have been executed so as to check the bodily energy, emotional well-being, and staying strength of the contributors. Kettlebells are significantly used these days in health gyms and endeavor centers. Due to the improvement of technology and advertising techniques, kettlebells in the interim are furthermore presented on line and can be shipped straight away to your private home.

Even YOU should buy kettlebells and do your private exercise workout routines at domestic effortlessly and luxury. If you are need to look and sense suitable, then I strongly recommend that you strive a few kettlebell sports sports and sporting sports.You will definitely provide you with notable results! Save some time and electricity with this very beneficial, comfortable, and effective device that might come up with confident best outcomes on your frame. If you would love to investigate extra approximately kettlebells and extra improtantly, experince them for yourself, I may want to encourage you to shop for one your self and start education at domestic.

"Training gives us an outlet for suppressed energies created via using stress and consequently tones the spirit truely as exercising conditions the body."

Arnold Schwarzenegger

Benefits of Kettlebell Training

Just like a few other fitness device, the number one reason of kettlebells is to create resistance on your muscles whilst the usage of them. With their alternatively easy but particular form, they'll be applied in a large sort of techniques. In your first enjoy with kettlebell training, you can experience turning into fatigued and sore speedy. Of route, it is everyday to revel in a chunk of higher degrees of pain and fatigue than normally in the path of or after your first kettlebell exercise exercises but as you still use them, each day or each one of a kind day, your muscles will get used to the pressure, and in the end, you will be capable of cope with more weight and flow longer without getting tired!

Weightlifting the use of kettlebells offers many notable advantages for your frame. Some benefits the kettlebell has to provide are:

1. Full body conditioning. Kettlebell schooling gives you a synchronized body workout that

trains your whole frame. From head to toe, the effects of kettlebell exercises can be seen and felt. Due the enormous sort of possible uses of the kettlebell, you may in truth experience the effects of the training in your muscle tissues, particularly on your, legs, hips, stomach place, and arms.

2. Physical power. Weightlifting and working out has exceptional one foremost position (except aesthetic advantages) developing your power. Training with kettlebells will increase your muscle strength and strength with out decreasing the mobility of your frame.

three. Endurance. Your schooling is prepared into one-of-a-kind exercise techniques, some of which increase your body persistence. It also can feature a cardio workout which permit's you pass longer without getting fatigued. Also, your muscular and joint density may even increase leaving them thicker and sturdier.

4. Enhanced frame mobility and coordination. Kettlebell exercising exercises, with their severa unique actions, will help you enhance you frame's mobility further to coordination.

5. Self self warranty. Workouts the use of kettlebells will in the end give you a more toned body which, in maximum instances, boosts one's self confidence.

6. Safe education. Most kettlebells are smaller than special training system. They are clean to deal with and provide you with a convenient and safe way to educate.

7. Comfortable and available. Kettlebells can be used and taken with you to nearly any palce your property, a park, your lawn, a health club and so on. The listing may want to pass on all the time. You may even maintain some to your automobile just so educate even as you're traveling.

eight. Calorie burning. Kettlebell training is taken into consideration as one of the exquisite processes to burn energy. According to the American Council on Exercise (ACE), exercising routines using kettlebells burn 20.2 electricity constant with minute! Over 1,2 hundred calories in step with hour! This is quite a exquisite range for individuals who desire to achieve a better body assemble faster.

Common Kettlebell Exercises

Different number one kettlebell sporting activities are indexed underneath at the side of the muscle groups they target and the benefits they carry.

Before doing any of the following carrying occasions, as you probable already understand, you have to warm your body up. Warming your muscle tissue and joints up will notably lessen the hazard of harm. If you start your exercise with out warming up first, your muscle companies and joints might be more prone to damage, you'll be worn out a bargain faster due to the muscle mass' unpreparedness to pressure.

When you are finished prepping for education, draw close your water packing containers and hand towels and located them with the useful resource of your trouble due to the fact you'll want them in the machine. Let's begin!

1. Kettlebell swing

The most easy of all kettlebell physical activities. One or two palms may be used on this ordinary. It works the hamstrings, glutes, stomach and lowerback, the top and middle once more, inclusive of the trapezius muscle beneath the neck.

Directions:

Stand in a squatting role. Knees bent. Then hold the kettlebell with one or each palms downward to the floor.

Raise the kettlebell then swing it beginning from your returned the usage of your hips. Hold the kettlebell on your arms at the identical time as straightening your lower once more.

Hold the kettlebell together with your hand however do not exert pressure out of your palms. Let your hips and legs do the art work.

Once you have got got straightened your back, your fingers want to now be perpendicular in your frame whilst preserving the kettlebell.

Finally, flow once more to the squatting position and repeat the steps for patterned repetitions

2. Kettlebell snatch

Usually the following important workout to examine after reading the swing. This is a totally technical workout that must be achieved effectively to achieve all of the advantage from it. It works the hamstrings, glutes, lower back muscle businesses, trapezius, deltoids, biceps, and triceps.

Directions:

Hold the kettlebell by way of the use of gripping it with one hand. Hold your hand close to one stop of the U-commonplace bar.

Just like the swing, begin via fame in a squat position, knees bent, and float the ball among your legs.

Move the ball upward and as it reaches the volume of your face, flick your wrist up sincerely so the kettlebell rests on your forearm and maintain raising the kettlebell until your arm is without a doubt vertical upward.

When your arm is vertically extended, the cycle repeats. But be cautious at the same time as reducing the ball and ensure to lower the ball the equal manner you lifted it to prevent any accidents.

three. Kettlebell easy and press

The technique for this workout is quite similar to the take maintain of, moreover with the flick of the wrist. But this time, in place of flicking your wrist at forehead height, flick your wrist at chest top. This exercise additionally has a very particular method to it and must be finished successfully. It works the deltoids, biceps, triceps, in addition to the better over again.

Directions:

Using the identical starting feature as the swing and the grab, in this workout you need to bend your knees and throw the kettlebell backwards.

When the kettlebell is ready to attain the peak of your shoulder, keep in mind to flick your wrist indoors making the kettlebell relaxation for your forearm beside your chest. Clean the kettlebell with the resource of bending your elbow absolutely.

Make sure to put your fingers in the the front of your chest and rest the cope with of the kettlebell among your index finger and your thumb

Chapter 11: Common Mistakes to Avoid

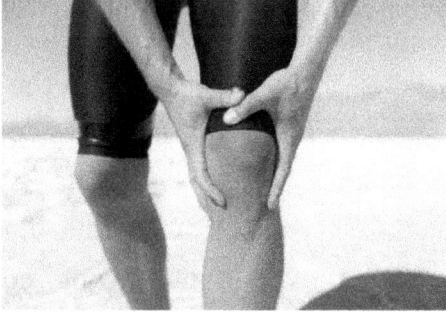

As, I already stated in advance, bypass-schooling and kettlebell training is one of the present day traits in health.However, due to their reputation, many humans are appearing kettlebell physical video games with wrong shape and techniques. Thus creating threat for damage and don't obtain all the blessings that they will get maintain of.

Here are a number of the maximum commonplace mistakes which are executed time and again once more with reference to bypass-training and kettlebell training.

Isolated Focus

It isn't clever to use kettlebells to do certainly one movement or attention on a unmarried muscle, like bicep curls.

The kettlebell is designed to region the center of the mass a long way from the body to enhance balance and strength. The kettlebell swing makes severa muscle tissue paintings and consequently will boom the coronary coronary heart charge which ends within the frame walking as a unmarried unit.

Listen for your Body

Always test your self earlier than, after and in some unspecified time in the destiny of exercising. Your frame will will let you recognise if some issue isn't right. All you want to do is pay hobby.

Wrist pain

Your wrists will excellent bruise and enjoy painful even as you are doing all of your easy smooth and press or clutch the wrong way.

Lower again pain

You need to be the usage of your lower decrease lower again in swinging the weight at the same time as you are bended on the waist; in location of letting your legs and hips do the paintings.

Don't confuse those signs and symptoms and signs with working and schooling tough.

Keep Score

Hitting a reason feels very profitable and fun. But how do you apprehend in case you're there or now not if you aren't measuring your results?

Perhaps you are someone who famous this to be tedious however that is one actvity that need to be finished. It will carry you greater consequences quicker.

I advise that you get a special mag wherein you jot down how many reps you've accomplished inside or how masses time it took you to get a positive WOD completed. Also record the weights which you used to your exercising workouts. This is optionally to be had but what I do is I jot down how I revel in in advance than and after the wrokout.

When "the rating" you'll recognise if you have emerge as more potent and quicker, and if you are shifting towards your desires or now not.

Have Direction

"A man without a goal is form of a deliver with out a rudder."

Thomas Carlyle

A mistake that many beginners make isn't always placing any dreams, as a end result having no route. You should continuously set desires with regards to workout and health.

Stick to a positive plan or health ordinary and results will come!

Useful suggestions to maintain in mind

Remember that it takes time to obtain everything. Kettlebell training isn't as clean as it sometimes seems. It requires staying strength, lengthy-time period strength of will, perspiration, willpower, and mental preparedness.

Here are a few tips for you:

A unique warmness-up to start your day. Warming up before you start doing all of your workout is the remarkable way to keep away from any damage at some point of the exercise. Shaking your muscle organizations and doing multiple repetitions of number one bodily video video games will assist put together your muscle tissue for what's coming.

Get a organisation grip at the address. Hold the kettlebell tightly while appearing unique sports and moves.

Have a cooldown consultation after your workout. I may strongly endorse which you have a brief "cooldown" proper after your exercise. It may be perfect for your cardiovascular system. To keep away from

DOMS (Delayed Onset Muscle Soreness), stretch your muscles and joints.

Perfect your swing. It might also seem like, on the same time as looking one of a kind people doing swings, they use their fingers to raise the kettlebells, but they aren't (as a minimum if they may be doing it efficaciously). In truth, the stress that makes the kettlebell flow comes from the hip and gluteal part of the frame. The hands are there to truely maintain the kettlebell in location. They do no longer exert any strain on the kettlebell. The force comes from status up and shifting your hips.

Some extra pointers for enhancing your swing:

You shouldn't stand to your ft. Keep your heels flat at the floor at the identical time as acting swings.

Keep your hips proper away whilst recognition and refrain from pushing your hips forward.

Raise the kettlebell up on your chin and now not higher. Be certain to growth your fingers even as swinging and allow the kettlebell flow into down on its private.

Set apart time for your sports. Hectic schedules and "all at once" appointments make it difficult to set aside time for a exercising. Always mark your exercise workout routines in your planners and schedules. Lack of time is regularly used as an excuse of now not working out. We've all heard human beings say "I'm too busy", "I don't have time for that", "My Schedule is packed." Yes, we frequently appear short of time however there's constantly a manner to squeeze in a short WOD some time in some unspecified time in the future of the day.

Momentum is essential on the subject of exercise continuously. There can be times that you'll be so prompted which you do your sporting events each single day, and consume healthy, and tell yourself time and again that you may do it. But there can be those activities if you need to throw you off the momentum that you have been building up. Self-manipulate is also a exercising you want to do. Pick your self up and get lower again in the sport.

Mix it up. Try a few detail new at the same time as the vintage workout workouts, sports and sports begin to enjoy stupid. Keep topics clean and interesting and to exercising with one in every of a type muscle businesses. You don't exchange your recurring every week, in reality shift it round a chunk.

Learn to love your habitual. If you're unmotivated and are not willing to do your exercising routine, it's much more likely that you'll give up and be left and no longer using a improvement the least bit. Just maintain at it. Every exercising desires practice and mastering. It isn't some thing you'll be an expert at within a few minutes. Start gradual at the begin, and don't push yourself too tough. For instance: on the primary day, do thirty pushups. On the following, add ten more.

Lastly reward your self. Rewards will help to keep you influenced. Never praise yourself with food, until you want to do your workout habitual all once more. Go to the spa, exit collectively along with your friends or go with the flow watch a movie. After all you deserve it!

Kettlebell WODs

Understanding the WODs

Example

Fran

Thruster ninety five lbs

Pull-ups

Instructions: Complete 21-15-9 reps of the sporting activities for time.

Explanation

This WOD is known as 'Fran'. It includes physical video games: a thruster with 95 lbs weight and pull-ups.

You need to complete 21 thrusters, 21 pull-ups, 15 thrusters, 15 pull-usaand 9 thrusters, nine pull-ups.

The reason of this workout is to finish the bodily video games as rapid as feasible. That method which you must time your results and document them every time you try this WOD. Those way you may have a look at your effects and see your improvement.

IMPORTANT: Don't forget approximately to warmness up earlier than the exercises to aviod harm!

Warning: The physical activities on this eBook are alleged to be used as a deliver of reference and WOD hints. Please talk with an authorized teacher on a way to carry out the carrying activities used in this eBook to keep away from harm. Visit www.CrossFit.Com for extra facts.

WOD #1

10 Clean-and-Jerks with KBs

Instructions: Perform 10 units of the exercise and relaxation 30 seconds in among the gadgets.

WOD #2

Repetition Snatches

Instructions: Perfrom as many reps as feasible in 3 mins (with each arm).

WOD #three

10 Heavy Swings

Instructions: Do 5-10 units of the exercising with 30 60 seconds relaxation in among.

WOD #four

1 air squat

1 lunge (each leg)

WOD #five

Two-exceeded KB swings

Instructions: Complete as many reps as you could inside 10 minutes.

WOD #6

20 Jump Squats

Instructions: Perform 20 bounce squats with a steady rythm. Do a total of eight-10 rounds for time.

WOD #7

15 kettlebell swings

10 goblet squats

Instructions: Do as many units as feasible indoors 10 mins without resting.

WOD #8

20 Swings

10 (9-8-7-6-five-four-three-2-1-0) Push-ups

Instructions: Do a complete of tens devices. Start with doing 20 KB swings and 10 Push-ups. With each next set, reduce the form of push u.S.By way of 1 till you reach zero.

WOD #9

eight Around the body passes (each guidelines)

12 Front Squats

12 KB Deadlifts

10 Swings (-passed)

6 Half get-ups (every element)

Instructions: Do 3 to 4 rounds of the sports as quick as you may.

WOD #10

12 Kettlebell Swings

10 Windmills

8 Kettlebell Swing Punches

20 Russian twists (every aspect)

12 Goblet Squats

Instructions: Complete 2-five gadgets as fast as you can.

WOD #11

10 kettlebell swings

5 facet plank rows with leg bring (each facet)

10 goblet plie squats

5 smooth & preses (every arm)

Instructions: Complete as many reps as feasible inside 15 mins.

WOD #12

One Handed Swing

Reverse Lunge

Overhead Clean

Squat & Press

Snatch

Clean, Squat & Press

Instructions: Do 1 minute of every factor of each workout. Rest 1 minute the various bodily activities.

WOD #13

Snatch

Press Ups

Double Handed Squats

Slow Mountain Climbers

Double Lunge

Instructions: Do every exercising for an c program languageperiod of 3 minutes. Rest inbetween the sporting activities for 1 minute.

WOD #14

Run 400m

Max push-ups

Max pull-ups

12 double Kettlebell press

Instructions: Complete a whole of 4 rounds. Record amount of push usaand pull-america of americadone.

WOD #15

20 squat flips

10 lateral lunges (every side)

10 push preses with KB (every thing)

Instructions: Perform as many gadgets as you can inside 15 mins.

WOD #16

One Handed Swing

Clean & Press

Side Lunge

Clean & Squat

Instructions: Perform 2 minute periods of every workout. Rest 1 minute amongst sporting events. Do to a few rounds.

WOD #17

five KB Deadlifts

five Push-ups

5 KB High Pulls

5 Push-ups

five Two-hand KB Swings

five Push-ups

5 Goblet Squats

5 Push-ups

Instructions: Do as many rounds as you could internal 20 mins.

WOD #18

25 burpees

45 one-arm KB swings (Righ side)

forty five one-arm KB swings (Left aspect)

25 burpees

Rest three mins

Instructions: Complete one to two rounds as speedy as you may.

WOD #19

10 Around-the-Body Passes

10-12 Bent Rows

10-12 Deadlifts

10 Figure 8's

5 Half Get-Up's

15-20 KB Swings

10-15 Front Squats

5-10 Windmills

Instructions: Do a complete of units as rapid as possible (resting among devices).

WOD #20

8 Windmills

10 Slingshots

8 Two-Handed Swings

five High Pulls

10 Lunge Presses

Instructions:Do to a few units of the carrying activities as rapid as you may.

WOD #21

15 Two Hand Swings

10 One Hand Swing s

10 One-Arm Clean and Push Presses

5 Bottoms-Up Cleans (each hand)

five Windmills (each hand)

10 Front Squats

50 Hand-to-Hand Swings

Instructions: Complete to a few units. Rest 30 to 45 seconds inbetween physical sports.

WOD #22

Swing

Double Lunge

High Pulls

Squat & Press

Snatch

Sit & Press

Instructions: Perform 1 minute of each workout for every issue. Between the sports activities, do 10 push-ups.

WOD #23

Three Rounds:

10 Body weight squats

five Alternate lunges (every leg)

5 Push-ups

Four Rounds:

20 Two-exceeded Swings

10 Kettlebell Twists

20 Kettlebell Thrusters

Chapter 12: Slow Mountain Climbers

Alternating Swing

Double Lunge

Prush Ups

Jumping Lunges

Dirty Dogs

Bob & Weave

High Pulls

Squat & Press

Instructions: Do 1 minute of each workout. For those wearing activities which want to be performed on each detail, do 1 minute on each difficulty. Rest 15 seconds between the sports activities.

WOD #30

10 Swings

6 Reverse Lunges (each issue)

10 Squat & Presses

12 Cleans

eight Press Ups

6 Sit & Presses

Instructions: Do to a few rounds of the carrying sports activities.

WOD #31

50 One Handed Swings

25 Snatches (each aspect)

25 Clean & Presses (each element)

25 Reverse Lunges (every component)

25 Squat & Presses (each element)

Instructions: Perform all sports activities sports as rapid as viable.

WOD #32

25 Snatches (each element)

25 Squat & Presses (each component)

25 High Pulls (every aspect)

25 Bob & Weaves (every issue)

50 One Handed Swings (every element)

Instructions: Perform all sporting sports as brief as viable.

WOD #33

10 KB Deadlifts

5 Push-ups

10 KB High Pulls

five Push-ups

10 Two-hand KB Swings

10 Goblet Squats

5 Push-ups

10 Goblet Squats

five Push-ups

Instructions: Do to three rounds as quickly as you may.

WOD #34

five Snatches

5 Squat & Press

5 Double Lunge

20 Double Handed Swings

10 Burpees

20 Fast Mountain Climbers

Instructions: Do as many rounds of the primary block of sports activities sports inside 7 minutes. Do as many rounds of the second one block internal 7 minutes too. Rest inside the various 2 block for 1 to 2 mins.

WOD #35

10 One Handed Swings

10 High Pulls

10 Snatches

10 Clean, Squat & Presses

Instructions: Complete six to eight rounds as quickly as you could.

WOD #36

One Handed Swings (each aspect)

Squat & Press (each side)

High Pulls (each facet)

Double Lunges (every side)

Instructions: Do 30 seconds of every exercise. Complete to three rounds. Rest 2 minutes amongst rounds.

WOD #37

Double Squat

Press Ups

Reverse Lunge

Burpees

Clean & Press

Instructions: Do every exercise for 1 minute. Rest 15 to 30 seconds some of the carrying sports. Do a complete of rounds.

WOD #38

Snatch (each aspect)

Clean & Press (each thing)

Burpee

Jump Squats

Windmill (each component)

Lunge & Hop (each detail)

Press Ups

Sit & Press

Instructions: Do every exercise for 1 minute. Rset for 15 seconds among sports activities.

WOD #39

6-10 KB Deadlifts

10 Push-ups

6 -10 KB High Pulls

8 Push-ups

6-10 Two-hand KB Swings

6 Push-ups

6-10 Goblet Squats

4 Push-ups

Instructions: Do as many rounds as you can within 20 mins.

WOD #forty

10 KB Deadlifts

10 Push-ups

10 KB High Pulls

10 Push-ups

10 Two-hand KB Swings

10 Goblet Squats

10 Push-ups

10 Push-ups

10 Goblet Squats

10 Push-ups

Instructions: Do as many rounds as you can interior 20 minutes.

WOD #41

Windmill

Squat & Press

Alternating Swings (every aspect)

Double Lunge

Instructions: Perform 2 minute intervals of every workout. Rest 1 minute amongst bodily games. Do to 3 rounds.

WOD #forty

3min capture (opposition weight)

1min relaxation

3min grasp (opposition weight)

1min rest

3min seize (competition weight)

3x static preserve jerks

Instructions:

WOD #43

5 Single Leg Deadlift

five Side Lunge

5 T Push Up

20 Double Handed Swings

20 No Kettlebell Reverse Lunges

20 No Kettlebell Squats

Instructions: Do as many rounds of the first block of physical video games inner 7 minutes. Do as many rounds of the second block interior 7 mins too. Rest in among the 2 block for 1 to 2 minutes.

WOD #forty 4

Double Handed Swing (every trouble)

Overhead Forward Lunge

Clean, Squat & Press

High Pulls

Instructions: Perform 2 minute durations of every exercising. Rest 1 minute between wearing activities. Do to a few rounds.

WOD #forty five

Snatch (each aspect)

Burpee

Push Ups

Alternating Swing

Overhead Press (each element)

Squat Thrusts

Instructions: Perform 1 minute periods of every exercise. Rest 15 seconds amongst bodily video games. Do three to 4 rounds.

WOD #forty six

10 Alternating Swings

10 Press Ups

10 High Pulls

10 Fast Mountain Climbers

10 Snatches

10 Jumping Lunges

Instructions: Complete 2 rounds as short as viable.

WOD #forty seven

10 One Handed Swings

10 High Pulls

10 Snatches

10 Clean & Presses

10 Alternating Swings

10 Squat & Presses

10 Side Lunges

10 Double Handed Swings

10 Reverse Lunge & Presses

Instructions: After every 3 wearing activities relaxation for 1 minute. Complete 2 rounds as speedy as you could.

WOD #48

10 One-hand swing smooth and jerks

10 One-hand swing snatches

10 Turkish get-ups

10 Side presses

10 One-hand excessive pulls

10 One-hand swings

10 Two-hand swings

10 Around frame passes

Instructions: Complete one spherical as rapid as feasible. Rest ninety seconds some of the sports activities activities.

WOD #40 nine

eight One-hand swing smooth and jerks

8 One-hand swing snatches

8 Turkish get-ups

8 Side presses

8 One-hand immoderate pulls

8 One-hand swings

8 Two-hand swings

8 Around frame passes

Instructions: Complete   rounds as fast as viable. Rest 30 60 seconds a number of the physical sports.

WOD #50

12 One-hand swing easy and jerks

12 One-hand swing snatches

12 Turkish get-ups

12 Side presses

12 One-hand excessive pulls

12 One-hand swings

12 Two-hand swings

12 Around body passes

Instructions: Complete three rounds as brief as possible. Rest 30 60 seconds the diverse physical video video games.

WOD #51

10 One-hand swing clean and jerks

10 Around body passes

10 One-hand swing snatches

10 Turkish get-ups

10 Side preses

10 One-hand high pulls

10 One-hand swings

10 Two-hand swings

Instructions: Complete to three devices. Rest 90 seconds among wearing sports.

WOD #fifty

Step-Out Swings

Windmills

Push Presses

High Pull Burpees

Spider Drags

Instructions: Do every exercising for an c program languageperiod of 30 seconds (in line with aspect for bodily activities that isolate every element). Complete or three rounds, with as many reps as you may.

WOD #53

6 Step-Out Swings

8 Windmills

6 Lunges

eight Push Presses

6 High Pull Burpees

8 Spider Drags

Instructions: Complete to a few rounds as fast as viable.

WOD #fifty four

3 pullups

10 pushups

15 air squats

10 single arm swings (every aspect)

200m run

Instructions: Do as many rounds as feasible interior 25 minutes.

WOD #fifty five

2 KB swings (one element only)

1 clean (one side satisfactory)

1 KB squat

2 push presses (one thing only)

Instructions: Do physical video video games 1,2 and 4 for one element only. Then do the subsequent spherical with the opposite arm. Do as many rounds as you can in this way.

WOD #56

nine unmarried-arm swings (each side)

5 place jumps

400m run

Instructions: Do as many roudns as you can interior 15 minutes.

WOD #fifty seven

20 (15-10-5) Double Handed Squats

20 (15-10-five) Snatches

20 (15-10-five) Reverse Lunges

20 (15-10-5) Push Ups

20 (15-10-5) Double Handed Swings

Instructions: Do 4 "countdown" units. Start with 20 reps for each workout, lowering the form of reps with the useful resource of five with every round.

WOD #fifty eight

Burpees

Slow Mountain Climbers

Alternating Swings

Press Ups

Double Handed Squats

Sit & Press

Double Handed Swings

Fast Mountain Climbers

Instructions: Do each exercising for an c program languageperiod of 30 seconds. Rest inbetween the sports activities activities for 30 seconds.

WOD #fifty nine

Kettlebell push press (each facet)

1 minute rest

Instructions: Do 2 minutes of every difficulty of the number one exercise. After that relaxation one minute

WOD #60

10 single arm KB swings (each aspect)

10 pushups

10 air squats

Instructions: Do as many rounds as you can inside 12 minutes.

WOD #61

five minute grab

Rest 5 mins

5 minute double arm jerk

Rest five mins

three minute take hold of

Rest three minutes

three minute double arm jerk

Rest three minutes

2 minute grasp

Rest 2 minutes

2 minute double arm jerk

Instructions: Do as many reps as possible of the given sports internal given time frames.

WOD #sixty

50 air squats

50 single arm swings (each arm)

50 push presses (every arm)

50 air squats

50 pushups

50 double arm swings

50 air squats

Instructions: Complete one spherical for time.

WOD #sixty 3

five container jumps

7 pushups

10 heavy double arm swings

Instructions: Do as many rounds as feasible inside 10 mins.

WOD #sixty four

1minute max burpees

3minute smooth and push press (Right problem)

1 minute max burpees

three minute clean and push press (Left facet)

1 minute max burpeesInstructions: Do as many reps of the sports as you may.

WOD #sixty 5

five KB push preses (one component)

10 KB unmarried arm swings (one aspect)

10 field jumps

Instructions: Do as many rounds as viable internal 12 minutes. Alternate aspects for sports activities 1 and 2 with each round.

WOD #66

6 single-arm swings (every element)

12 walking lunges

6 push press (each difficulty)

Instructions: Do as many rounds as you can inner 15 minutes.

WOD #67

7 One-exceeded Kettlebell Swings (7 reps each issue)

10 KB Push-Ups

12 KB Cleans

eight KB Deadlifts

Instructions: Complete 4 to five rounds as fast as you can.

WOD #sixty eight

6 One Handed Swings (each hand)

8 Reverse Lunges (every leg)

6 Overhead Cleans

6 Squat & Presses

eight Snatches

6 Clean, Squat & Presses

Instructions: Complete a whole of to three rounds for time.

WOD #69

12 KB High Pulls (every hand)

10 Two-Handed KB Swings

8 Windmills (each facet)

8 KB Rows

Instructions: Complete three to 5 rounds as fast as you may.

WOD #70

5 Clean, Squat & Press

5 Double Lunge

5 T Push Ups

8 Burpees

20 Jumping Lunges

20 Double Handed Swings

Instructions: Do as many rounds of the primary block of bodily video games indoors 7 mins. Do as many rounds of the second block internal 7 mins too. Rest in a few of the 2 block for 1 to two minutes.

WOD #71

eight Burpees

6 Double Lunges

8 Clean & Presses

8 Jump Squats

6 Windmills

6 Single Leg Deadlifts

Instructions: Do 3 to five units as short as you may.

WOD #seventy two

Two Hand Swings

One Hand Swings

One-Arm Clean and Push Presses

Bottoms-Up Cleans (each hand)

Windmills (every hand)

Front Squats

Hand-to-Hand Swings

Instructions: Perform 1 minute durations of the bodily sports. Relaxation 1 minute the various sports activities. Complete as many reps as you could.

WOD #seventy three

12 Burpees

eight Slow Mountain Climbers

6 Alternating Swings (each trouble)

8 Sit & Presses

10 Double Handed Swings

8 Press Ups

10 Double Handed Squats

10 Fast Mountain Climbers

Instructions: Do to three gadgets as quick as feasible.

WOD #seventy four

8 Alternating KB Rows (every side)

6 Windmills (each factor)

eight KB High Pulls

Chapter 13: One Hundred Pull-Ups

a hundred Push-ups

a hundred Sit-ups

100 Squats

Goal: Complete inside the shortest amount of time viable.

Instructions: Complete all repetitions of every exercise in advance than shifting to the following.

Annie

Double-unders

Sit-ups

Goal: Complete for time.

Instructions: 50-40-30-20 and 10 rep rounds.

Barbara

20 Pull-ups

30 Push-ups

40 Sit-ups

50 Squats

Goal: Complete for time.

Instructions: Complete a total of 5 rounds and time every of them. Rest precisely three minutes among every spherical.

Chelsea

five Pull-ups

10 Push-ups

15 Squats

Goal: Complete for rounds.

Instructions: Each minute on the minute for 30 min.

Cindy

five Pull-ups

10 Push-ups

15 Squats

Goal: Complete as many rounds as feasible in 20 min.

Instructions: Complete as many rounds of the sports activities listed as possible, within 20 mins.

Diane

Deadlift 225 lbs

Handstand push-ups

Goal: Complete for time.

Instructions: 21-15-9 reps

Elizabeth

Clean a hundred thirty 5 lbs

Ring Dips

Goal: Complete for time.

Instructions: Complete 21-15-nine reps of every physical activities as quick as viable.

Eva

Run 800 meters

2 pood KB swing, 30 reps

30 pullups

Goal: Complete for time.

Instructions: Complete five rounds of these 3 sports.

Fran

Thruster ninety five lbs

Pull-ups

Goal: Complete for time.

Instructions: Complete 21-15-nine reps of the sports activities activities.

Grace

Clean and Jerk one hundred thirty 5 lbs

Goal: Complete for time.

Instructions: Complete 30 reps of the exercise for time.

Helen

4 hundred meter run

1.Five pood Kettlebell swing x 21

Pull-america12 reps

Goal: Complete for time.

Instructions: Complete 3 rounds for time

Isabel

Snatch a hundred thirty five kilos

Goal: whole for time.

Instructions: 30 reps of the workout for time

Jackie

1000 meter row

Thruster 45 lbs (50 reps)

Pull-ups (30 reps)

Goal: Complete for time.

Instructions: Complete all repetitions of every workout earlier than transferring to the subsequent.

Karen

Wall-ball 100 fifty pics

Goal: Complete for time.

Instructions: Do 100 fifty Wall-Ball pictures for time.

Kelly

Run 4 hundred meters

30 box bounce, 24 inch area

30 Wall ball photographs, 20 pound ball

Goal: Complete for time

Instructions: Complete 5 rounds for time.

Linda

Deadlift 1 half BW

Bench BW

Clean three/four BW

Goal: Complete for time.

Instructions: 10/nine/8/7/6/5/four/three/2/1 rep rounds for time.

Lynne

Bodyweight bench press (e.G., equal amount on bar as you weigh)

Pullups

Goal: 5 rounds for optimum reps.

Instructions: Complete five rounds and do as many reps as viable. Three is No time detail to this WOD.

Mary

five Handstand push-ups

10 1-legged squats

15 Pull-ups

Goal: Complete as many rounds as feasible interior time frame.

Instructions: Complete as many rounds of the sports activities as feasible inner 20 min.

Nancy

four hundred meter run

Overhead squat ninety 5 lbs x 15

Goal: Complete for time

Instructions: Complete 5 rounds for time

Nicole

Run 4 hundred meters

Max rep Pull-ups

Goal: Complete as many rounds as viable in 20 minutes.

Instructions: Complete as many rounds as viable in 20 minutes and record quantity of pull-u.S.A.Finished for every round.

"Hero" WODs

Since it's early days, this unique fitness utility has supported the men and women in uniform. It honors the heroes who've died protecting our lives and our nations.

The hero WODs are the most excessive workout workouts that you may enjoy. They are designed to be very intense in honor of the fallen heroes.

Adrian

three Forward rolls

five Wall climbs

7 Toes to bar

9 Box jumps, 30" situation

Goal: Complete for time.

Instructions: Complete 7 rounds as brief as feasible.

Arbate

Run 1 mile

one hundred fifty five pound Clean and jerk, 21 reps

Run 800 meters

155 pound Clean and jerk, 21 reps

Run 1 Mile

Goal: Complete for time.

Instructions: Complete all sporting sports and movements as speedy as viable.

Brehm

15 foot Rope climb, 10 ascents

225 pound Back squat, 20 reps

30 Handstand push-ups

Row 40 electricity

Goal: Complete for time.

Instructions: Complete all bodily activities as fast as viable.

Bulger

Run a hundred fifty meters

7 Chest to bar pull-ups

130 5 pound Front squat, 7 reps

7 Handstand push-ups

Goal: Complete for time.

Instructions: Complete 10 rounds as rapid as possible.

Carse

ninety five pound Squat smooth

Double-under

185 pound Deadlift

24" Box leap

Begin every spherical with a 50 meter Bear flow slowly.

Goal: Complete for time.

Instructions: Do 21-18-15-12-nine-6-3 reps of the sports activities sports.

Daniel

50 Pull-ups

4 hundred meter run

ninety five pound Thruster, 21 reps

800 meter run

95 pound Thruster, 21 reps

4 hundred meter run

50 Pull-ups

Goal: Complete for time.

Instructions: Complete the sports activities activities as quick as possible.

Danny

24" subject leap, 30 reps

115 pound push press, 20 reps

30 pull-ups

Goal: Complete as many rounds indoors time body.

Instructions: Complete as many rounds as feasible inner 20 minutes.

Helton

Run 800 meters

30 reps, 50 pound dumbbell squat cleans

30 Burpees

Goal: Complete for time.

Instructions: Complete 3 rounds as brief as feasible.

Holbrook

115 pound Thruster, 5 reps

10 Pull-ups

a hundred meter Sprint

Rest 1 minute

Goal: Complete for time.

Instructions: Complete 10 rounds as short as possible.

Holleyman

five Wall ball pictures, 20 pound ball

three Handstand push-ups

225 pound Power smooth, 1 rep

Goal: Complete for time.

Instructions: Complete 30 rounds of the sports activities sports for time.

Hortman

Run 800 meters

eighty Squats

8 Muscle-ups

Goal: AMRAP in 45 min.

Instructions: Complete as many reps as viable inner 45 minutes.

JAG 28

Run 800 meters

28 Kettlebell swings, 2 pood

28 Strict Pull-ups

28 Kettlebell easy and jerk, 2 pood every

28 Strict Pull-ups

Run 800 meters

Goal: Complete for time.

Instructions: Complete bodily sports as short as possible.

Joshie

forty pound Dumbbell seize, 21 reps, right arm

21 L Pull-ups

forty pound Dumbbell take hold of, 21 reps, left arm

21 L Pull-ups

Goal: Complete for time.

Instructions: Complete three rounds for time. Note The snatches are complete squat snatches.

Ring dips

Push-ups

Goal: Complete for time

Instructions: 21-15-nine reps for time.

Lumberjack 20

20 Deadlifts (275lbs)

Run 400m

20 KB swings (2pood)

Run 400m

20 Overhead Squats (115lbs)

Run 400m

20 Burpees

Run 400m

20 Pullups (Chest to Bar)

Run 400m

20 Box jumps (24")

www.ingramcontent.com/pod-product-compliance
Lightning Source LLC
Chambersburg PA
CBHW051726020426
42333CB00014B/1166